WILDERNESS MEDICAL SOCIETY
Practice Guidelines
for Wilderness Emergency Care

WILDERNESS MEDICAL SOCIETY

Practice Guidelines for Wilderness Emergency Care

Fifth Edition

Edited by William W. Forgey, MD

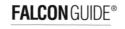

GUILFORD, CONNECTICUT
HELENA, MONTANA
AN IMPRINT OF THE GLOBE PEQUOT PRESS

To buy books in quantity for corporate use
or incentives, call **(800) 962–0973, ext. 4551,**
or e-mail **premiums@GlobePequot.com.**

A FALCON GUIDE®

Copyright © 1987, 1989, 1995, 2001, 2006 by Wilderness Medical Society

All rights reserved. No part of this book may be reproduced or transmitted in any form by any means, electronic or mechanical, including photocopying and recording, or by any information storage and retrieval system, except as may be expressly permitted by the 1976 Copyright Act or by the publisher. Requests for permission should be made in writing to The Globe Pequot Press, P.O. Box 480, Guilford, Connecticut 06437.

Falcon and FalconGuide are registered trademarks of Morris Book Publishing, LLC.

Text design: Lesley Weissman-Cook

Library of Congress Cataloging-in-Publication Data

Wilderness Medical Society.
  Wilderness Medical Society practice guidelines for wilderness emergency care / edited by William W. Forgey. — 5th ed.
    p. ; cm.
  ISBN-13: 978-0-7627-4102-1
  ISBN-10: 0-7627-4102-3
  1. Mountaineering injuries. 2. First aid in illness and injury. 3. Wilderness survival. 4. Medical emergencies. I. Forgey, William W., 1942- . II. Title. III. Title: Practice guidelines for wilderness emergency care.
    [DNLM: 1. Emergencies—Practice Guideline. 2. Emergency Treatment—Practice Guideline. 3. Recreation—Practice Guideline. 4. Travel—Practice Guideline. 5. Wounds and Injuries—therapy—Practice Guideline.   WB 105 W673w 2006]
  RC88.9.M6W54 2006
  616.02'5—dc22

                                                                        2006010025

Manufactured in the United States of America
Fifth Edition/First Printing

The authors and The Globe Pequot Press assume no liability for
accidents happening to, or injuries sustained by, readers who engage
in the activities described in this book.

Contents

Foreword

The Wilderness Medical Society Practice Guidelines are written for physician use at the generalist level. Many specialists (such as anesthesiologists, cardiovascular surgeons, and orthopedists) may well diagnose conditions and determine that more aggressive measures are indicated in certain circumstances and that they have the means to achieve them. The guidelines propose the best methodology for handling prehospital care for illness and injury occurring in wilderness areas. These protocols do not form the legal basis for training nonphysicians, although many of the techniques discussed have been incorporated into various proprietary wilderness first aid (WFA), wilderness first responder (WFR), and EMT-W training programs. The standardizations or legalization of these courses is not the purview of this document.

The first version of the *Wilderness Medical Society Practice Guidelines* (published as "position papers") was published in July 1987 as an insert in the society's newsletter. It encompassed eight topics, namely: CPR, medical evacuation, helicopter evacuation, hypothermia, high-altitude illness, snakebite, field water disinfection, and oral fluid and electrolytes. There were twenty-three authors cited, all of whom are acknowledged in the author list that follows.

The second edition was expanded to fifteen topics. This document was published as an insert in the society newsletter in 1989, under the editorship of Ken Iserson and with thirteen authors (also cited in the author list). These first two editions included levels of care, with different techniques being prescribed for non-EMT-, EMT-, and physician-level responders.

Levels of care were removed from the third iteration of this project, published in 1995 by ICS Books (now The Globe Pequot Press, the current publisher). Expanded to twenty-three topics, this edition also included the results of the Wilderness Medical Society Prehospital Committee study prepared by its members, E. Otten (Chair), W. Bowman, P. Hackett, M. Spadafora, and D. Tauber. This report, titled "Wilderness Prehospital Emergency Care (WPHEC) Curriculum" was a model curriculum, the components of which it was hoped would be extracted for various levels of prehospital wilderness medical training.

The society published the fourth edition of its guidelines (labeled the second edition by the publisher, The Globe Pequot Press) in 2001. Three new topics had been added: wilderness eye injuries, botanical encounters (contact and ingestion issues), and marine envenomations and poisonings.

This, the fifth edition of the Wilderness Medical Society guidelines, presents what the WMS Panel of Expert Reviewers feels is the best approach for the management of remote-area injuries and illness. This edition nudges the guidelines toward evidence-based medicine, with category stratification of its recommendations. The following criteria have been implemented:

- Category 1A: Strongly recommended for implementation and strongly supported by well-designed experimental, clinical, or epidemiological studies.
- Category 1B: Strongly recommended for implementation and supported by some experimental, clinical, or epidemiological studies and a strong theoretical rationale.
- Category 2: Suggested for implementation and supported by suggestive clinical or epidemiological studies or a theoretical rationale.
- Category 3: No recommendation. Conflicting or inadequate support by published articles. Frequently this information is included in a controversy section.

This material is published by the society for the use of its physician members. It is felt that much of this material is appropriate for inclusion in lay instructional courses. This edition does include significant input from the leadership of many of the commercial prehospital care providers. For their help, the editor is grateful. In the editor's opinion, their continued cooperation in an attempt to standardize and eventually gain legal acceptance of these courses would be in the public's best interest.

The following persons either contributed directly to the writing or were involved with the review, of previous editions, of these *Practice Guidelines*.

Col. Robert Allen, MD, USAF	William Forgey, MD
Wayne Askew, MD	Luanne Freer, MD
Paul S. Auerbach, MD, MS	Edward Geehr, MD
Howard Backer, MD	Gordon Giesbrecht, PhD
Richard Banta, MD	Paul Gill Jr., MD
Warren Bowman, MD	J. Richard Gorham, PhD
Capt. Frank Butler, MD, USN	Philip Goodman, MD
Michael Cardwell	Melissa Gray, EMT-1/C
Keith Conover, MD	Colin Grissom, MD
Lily Conrad, MD	Peter Hackett, MD
Richard Dart, MD	R. Scott Hammond, MD
Fred Darvill Jr., MD	William J. Henry, MD
Anne Dickison, MD	Bruce Holmstead
Steve Donelan	Kenneth Iserson, MD
Blair Erb, MD	David E. Johnson, MD
John Feagin Jr., MD	Linda Lindsey, RN

David Linn, MD
Michael Mackan, MD
Sherman A. Minton, MD
James Mohle, MD
Karl Neuman, MD
Edward Otten, MD
Bruce C. Paton, MD
Ian Rogers, MBBS
Matthew Russell, MD
Ramon Ryan, MD
Tod Schimelpfenig, EMT-1/C

Robert Schoene, MD
Joseph Serra, MD
James Shuler, MS, DO
Jay Skidmore, MD
Daniel Spaite, MD
John Sullivan, MD
Stephanie Thompson, MD
Buck Tilton, MS, EMT-W
David Townes, MD, MPH
Eric A. Weiss, MD
Ken Zafren, MD

Contributors to the current edition are:

Col. Robert Allen, MD, USAF
Capt. Brad L. Bennett, PhD, USN,
   NREMT-P, WEMT
Jolie Bookspan, PhD
Capt. Frank Butler, MD, USN
Steve Donelan, EMT-W
Luanne Freer, MD
Gordon Giesbrecht, PhD
Colin Grissom, MD
Murray Hamlet, DVM
David E. Johnson, MD
Lee Kaplan, MD

R. William Mackie, MD
Edward Otten, MD
Marshall Pitts, MD
Philip C. Rasori, MD
Ian Rogers, MBBS
Ben Rosner, MD, PhD
Tod Schlemelpfinig, EMT
Alton Thygerson, PhD
Buck Tilton, MS, EMT-W
Jim Wilkerson, MD
Robert Williams, MD
Ken Zafren, MD

Material in these guidelines is also contained in the *Wilderness Medicine Educational Lecture Series,* available as a Microsoft PowerPoint slide set and study guide published on CD by the society.

Authorization of the publication of these guidelines was under the auspices of the Board of Directors of the Wilderness Medical Society.

Copies of the Curriculum Vitae of the contributors are available from the society headquarters.

The editor is particularly grateful for the many members of the Wilderness Medical Society who have continued to demonstrate an active interest in contributing to these guidelines and to the support of the Wilderness Medical Society.

William W. Forgey, MD
Editor, *WMS Practice Guidelines*
Past President, Wilderness Medical Society

CHAPTER

Wilderness Evacuation

Recommendations are considered Category 1B by the WMS Panel of Expert Reviewers.

I. GENERAL INFORMATION

The mode and urgency of the evacuation should be appropriate for the problem. Calling for on-site evacuation (e.g., helicopter) versus evacuating a patient to care by foot or on a litter is decided upon in view of multiple factors, including:

- Severity of the illness or injury, including the psychological condition of the victim
- Rescue and medical skills of the rescuers
- Physical/psychological condition of the rescuers
- Availability of equipment and/or aid for the rescue
- Danger/difficulty of extracting the victim(s) by the various means available
- Time, a product of distance, terrain, weather (and the possible deterioration of the weather), and multiple other variables
- Cost

An evacuation deemed necessarily "urgent" considers the patient's life or significant morbidity to be at immediate risk. These guidelines indicate "nonurgent" evacuation in cases where the patient requires further evaluation and treatment but is not at immediate risk for significant morbidity or death.

Party leaders must know the capabilities of rescue organizations in the area the group is using and how to contact those organizations. All wilderness leaders must leave trip plans with a responsible person who can act on the group's behalf. If rescue by an outside group (rather than self-rescue by the party) has been determined to be the best course of action, the earlier it is initiated, the better. Waiting may allow deterioration of the patient and may jeopardize the entire rescue operation.

When requesting outside assistance, delayed response time, the safety of incoming rescuers, number of personnel responding, time to assemble, their time commitment, and the cost of the rescue must be considered. It is important to note that the safety of the rescuers or the group takes precedence over ideal management of the patient. Optimally, the entire group, including the patient, must make evacuation decisions.

In general, it is appropriate to postpone further travel and/or initiate evacuation from the wilderness for any person who has the following:

- Sustained or progressive physiological deterioration, manifested by orthostatic dizziness, syncope, tachycardia, bradycardia, dyspnea, altered mental status, progressive or significant weakness, or intractable vomiting and/or diarrhea; inability to tolerate oral fluids; or the return of loss of consciousness following head injury. In other words, if patients are not improving, they must get out!
- Debilitating pain.
- Inability to sustain travel at a reasonable pace due to a medical problem.
- Sustained abdominal pain with or without the passage of blood by mouth or rectum (not from an obviously minor source).
- Signs and symptoms of serious high-altitude illness.
- Infections that progress for more than twenty-four hours despite the administration of appropriate treatment.
- Chest pain that is not clearly originating from a minor musculoskeletal injury.
- The development of a psychological status that impairs the safety of the person or the group.
- Large or serious wounds, or wounds with complications (e.g., open fracture, gunshot wounds, deformed fractures, fractures impairing circulation, impaled objects, suspected spinal injury, certain burns as indicated in chapter 7).

Travel may continue if it is toward definitive care in the case of points 3, 4, and 8, or when descending in the case of point 5. This is understandably a general list, and specific comments on relevant medical concerns are made in the chapters that follow.

II. GUIDELINES FOR GROUND EVACUATION

If the decision has been made for a member of the party to walk out to obtain definitive care, the individual must not go alone unless there is no other alternative. Whenever possible, at least two members of the party, who are mentally and physically equipped to do so, must accompany the patient.

If anything more complex than a simple walkout of the patient is required, e.g., a litter carry, an on-site leader must be identified who will assume responsibility for the evacuation. If an outside rescue is to be requested, a decision must be made on the most efficacious method of requesting this help. A request for help is often exercised via electronic communication, e.g., a cell phone, but in all cases the request should be written first to ascertain inclusion of all the relevant information. The written request should include an assessment of the patient, of the situation (to include equipment, personnel, food, water), and a detailed location (map preferred) of the patient. The note should also include potential hazards to rescuers, limitations for vehicles, etc. Experience has shown that taking the time to write out a detailed note actually decreases total evacuation time. In assessing the anticipated length of evacuation time, the note must include the expertise and rescue experience of the persons in the field with the victim. In many countries a method of payment must be indicated before a rescue will be made. Without electronic communication, a written request for assistance will be hand-carried out by one member, but preferably two or three members, of the party.

During a litter evacuation, at least four (preferably six) bearers must handle the litter at all times, except when physically impossible, such as carries over a narrow bridge. Additional personnel must be available to relieve those handling the litter. The number of litter carriers will ideally be eight persons per 100 meters of travel over rough terrain and six persons per 100 meters over reasonably smooth trail. A total of eighteen litter carriers are required for the safest management of the litter over an extended distance. It is very demanding to carry a loaded litter for more than fifteen to twenty minutes without rotating porters or a significant break. Litter carries, especially over rugged terrain, can be agonizingly slow. One bearer will be in charge of the litter, directing lifting and moving, directing the passing of the litter over obstacles, and assuming responsibility for continuously monitoring and reassuring the patient. Many teams standardize the position at the left front of the litter as the litter "driver's" position. It is best to support a litter skeletally by utilizing straps, webbing, or pack frames rather than depending on hand grips.

The patient must be carefully "packaged" in the litter for maximum safety and comfort. Protect the patient's head and eyes. Pad stress points (e.g., where the straps press against the body) and the voids (e.g., in the small of the back and behind the knees). Protect from wind, cold, and precipitation. To prevent decubitus ulcers, have the patient move occasionally or alter the patient's position at least every two hours if he or she is unconscious. Expect to handle urine and fecal elimination by allowing the functional patient to leave the stretcher with assistance (if serious spine injuries can be cleared), or provide appropriate tilting and/or cleansing toweling to catch excrement. To prevent deep vein thrombosis it is necessary to allow leg movement or to move or massage legs hourly, as long as this does not increase the severity of the original injury. If the litter is improvised, test the system and padding first on an uninjured person.

III. GUIDELINES FOR HELICOPTER EVACUATION

Helicopters can significantly reduce the time to definitive care when used for emergency transportation of the sick or injured. The decision to use a helicopter for an evacuation must take into account clinical, logistical, and environmental factors. Using a helicopter always adds an element of risk both to rescuers and victim, and a note requesting an air evacuation should include all known specific hazards relative to the rescue. This risk must be balanced against the risk to the patient, other members of the party, or the rescue team if the patient is evacuated by ground. Evacuate by helicopter only if:

■ A victim's life will be saved.
■ The victim has a significantly better chance for full recovery via a helicopter evacuation.
■ The pilot believes that conditions are safe enough to do the evacuation.
■ A ground evacuation may be unusually dangerous to the ground crew.
■ Ground evacuation would be excessively prolonged.
■ There are not enough rescuers available for a ground evacuation.
   Four important points must be kept in mind:
■ It may be faster to evacuate a patient by ground rather than wait for a helicopter (especially in high-risk flight conditions).
■ The patient will need to be evacuated by ground if the helicopter is not able to respond, or if removal from the accident site would benefit the patient (e.g., descent for altitude sickness).
■ The patient may need to be moved to an appropriate landing site.
■ Do not use a helicopter to recover a corpse under emergency conditions.

A. Aircraft limitations

Helicopters have various configurations, with different capabilities and different crew skill levels. All helicopters are adversely affected by increased altitude, high environmental temperature, high wind, and heavy payload. The aircraft pilot makes the ultimate decisions concerning flight operations. A helicopter must not fly into known icing conditions or into even moderate storm conditions. Winds more than 45 mph, night flights into mountains, and landing in high winds are extremely hazardous. Not all helicopters or pilots are capable of flying by instruments into cloudy or foggy conditions. Moreover, instrument flight rules (IFR) are generally used only for airport-to-airport transport, not in flights to wilderness destinations, and most EMS helicopters are not equipped for IFR. Party leaders must be familiar with ground-to-air signals, and if radio communication is available, the ground crew must keep the helicopter crew updated on weather and other related conditions at the scene.

   Landing and taking off are the two most dangerous activities for both the air and ground crews. As altitude increases, the ability to make vertical hovers and land in small areas is greatly reduced. The optimal landing zone (LZ) is large, well marked, and relatively flat with a slope dropping slightly away from the LZ, and it has no tall objects on the perimeter and no loose debris that could be thrown up by the rapidly spinning blades. Marking at an LZ is best done with green reflective material and second best with red. The LZ may have to be prepared by the on-site personnel. It must be far enough from the patient so any maneuvering by the helicopter does not put the patient at risk. If there is no suitable landing zone, helicopters equipped for short haul or winch operations may be used.

The on-site personnel handling the patient must have some familiarity with helicopter operations. Helicopter landing zones are dangerous places. It is imperative to keep all nonessential personnel away from the area. If possible, assign personnel to keep a safe perimeter around the landing zone and to prevent people from approaching the craft. Wind generated by the helicopter is tremendous, and all ground personnel must protect themselves when the aircraft lands and takes off. In winter the wind chill from the rotor blades can cause rapid frostbite to areas of exposed skin. Never approach a helicopter until a signal has been given by one of the aircraft personnel. Never approach a helicopter from the rear, where the spinning tail rotor is invisible and therefore dangerous, unless it is a rear-entry aircraft and the safe-approach signal has been clearly understood. Once the helicopter is on the ground, all directions from the aircraft crew must be followed explicitly.

B. Airmedical considerations

The mechanics and physiology of flight must be understood if it is to be safely used for patient transport. Noise and vibration levels are high, and it may be difficult to monitor or even communicate with the patient in flight without special equipment. Helicopter cabins are not pressurized. Atmospheric and oxygen pressure go down as the aircraft goes up. Supplemental oxygen must be available for all patients. Medical devices with air bladders—e.g., MAST (military anti-shock trousers), air splints, and endotracheal tubes—must be monitored for overinflation. Ground transport may be a safer alternative for patients with a suspected pneumothorax, decompression sickness, or air embolism.

IV. CONTROVERSIES

Do wilderness travelers have a "right" to be rescued?

In the United States, it is often assumed that a cry for help will bring an immediate response, free of charge. There is, however, no guarantee that a rescue will be initiated, free or otherwise, despite the concerns of family and friends, the pressure of the media, and the availability of eager and willing rescuers. Evacuations from the wilderness create risk for the rescuers—who must walk in or fly in—and are typically very expensive. Search and rescue managers have to make tough decisions based on numerous factors, and the condition of the patient is only one of these factors. It is improper, therefore, to ask for help out of convenience when a group could carry out a self-rescue. Request assistance as a last resort, when life or limb is threatened, or when the group is unable to carry out their own rescue.

2

Myocardial Infarction, Acute Coronary Syndromes, and CPR

Recommendations are considered Category 1B by the WMS Panel of Expert Reviewers.

I. GENERAL INFORMATION

Acute Coronary Syndrome (ACS), including myocardial infarction and unstable angina, is a major cause of mortality. Chest pain is the most common reason for emergency calls to the U.S. Coast Guard and is the most common reason for EMS dispatch in the United States. In urban areas, approximately 15 percent of EMS transports for chest pain are due to documented ACS; in more rural areas, such as Scandinavia, up to 30 percent of chest-pain victims arriving to hospital by EMS transport have ACS. In the United States, mortality from ACS rises proportionally with the distance a victim lives from a CCU. In the predefibrillator era, mortality from myocardial infarction was 50 percent. In the years after defibrillators were available, but before thrombolytics were routinely used, acute mortality from ACS was approximately 15 to 20 percent and was improved mainly due to the routine use of aspirin, beta-blockers, and nitrates. In the post-thrombolytic era, mortality fell to 5 to 10 percent. With the advent of angioplasty for ACS, acute mortality in tertiary referral hospitals in the United States approaches 3 to 5 percent, and in Europe remains 5 to 7 percent. It is now recognized that arterial pathology with platelet-rich thrombii and inflamed, ulcerative plaque is the same in unstable angina as in myocardial infarction, only the extent of coronary flow obstruction is different. Immediate evacuation saves lives in the setting of ACS. The quickest route to the hospital is the best route, even if the victim has to walk at a slow pace. Physical rest is preferred, but if litter transport is impossible due to terrain or lack of assistance, the victim should attempt slow self-rescue. Reperfusion therapy, even up to thirty-six hours post-infarction, will reduce long-term mortality and complications from infarction. Death occurs from arrhythmias (bradycardic or tachycardic), shock (with or without pulmonary edema), or stroke. Even in settings far from medical help, simple measures can reduce mortality while the evacuation proceeds.

A. Recognition of acute coronary syndromes

1. Symptoms

a. Chest pain with or without radiation to the arm or jaw.

– Unstable angina pain will wax and wane and may be relieved by nitroglycerin. Pain radiating to the back or stomach suggests inferior myocardial infarction (MI). MI pain will not be completely relieved by nitrates.

b. Nausea with both anterior and inferior MI. When associated with diarrhea is usually a sign of impending shock with inferior MI and represents vagal shock.

c. Shortness of breath usually represents acute anterior MI or acute lateral MI with acute mitral regurgitation.

d. Diaphoresis, which is present with both anterior and inferior infarctions.

2. Signs

a. Blood pressure: A nonpalpable pulse indicates shock and usually correlates with systolic BP below 80 mmHg. If the victim has a palpable pulse in the standing position, then BP is usually over 80 mmHg systolic.

b. Heart rate: Above 100/minute is a sign of impending shock and anterior infarction. Pulse below 50/minute is a sign of inferior and often right ventricular infarction.

c. PVCs or PACs usually are signs of ischemia or infarction and occur early in course of ACS.

d. Syncope with sudden bradycardia: Sign of heart block and inferior and right venticular infarction.

e. Accelerated normal rhythm at 100–120/minute (lasting minutes) developing as pain improves is a good sign and indicates spontaneous coronary reperfusion.

3. Pathophysiology of coronary blood flow

a. Anterior infarction (LAD) vs. inferior infarction (right coronary) occlusions

– LAD flow occurs predominately in diastole and depends on diastolic BP to support flow.

– Slowing heart rate improves LAD flow and the proportion of time spent in diastole and will reduce infarct size and extent of ischemia.

– RCA flow occurs predominately in systole and depends on systolic BP for support of flow.

– Hypotension and excessive bradycardia will worsen RCA flow and may aggravate inferior infarction. Syncope after nitrate use indicates right ventricular infarction.

b. Coronary thrombus: present in nearly all patients with ACS. Dehydration, hypoxia, increased sympathetic output, catecholamine, fear, and exertion will increase platelet activation.

– Platelet receptor blockade will reduce likelihood of transmural MI in unstable angina and will reduce risk of reinfarction following spontaneous thrombolysis.

– Twenty-five percent of all transmural infarction patients will undergo spontaneous coronary thrombolysis and reperfusion in twenty-four hours.

c. Collateral flow: present to at least a slight extent in all patients; degree of collateral is related to the likelihood of improved outcome following transmural MI with complete coronary occlusion.

– Nitrates improve collateral flow, reduce venous return, and hence reduce subendocardial diastolic pressure and reduce infarction size and symptoms of ischemia.

d. Myocardial infarction is irreversible coronary ischemia leading to cell death.

e. Coronary ischemia is caused by an imbalance between myocardial oxygen supply and demand. The major determinants of myocardial oxygen demand are heart rate, BP (afterload), and myocardial contractility.

f. The major determinants of myocardial oxygen supply are coronary blood flow (related to coronary perfusion pressure, diastolic LV and RV wall pressure, and right atrial pressure) and partial pressure of coronary arterial oxygen and blood oxygen content.

B. Oral medications to reduce infarction size and improve mortality

The American Heart Association and American College of Cardiology (AHA/ACC) guidelines for acute myocardial infarction and unstable angina list four oral medications as having Class I indications for reduction in mortality and morbidity in the setting of ACS. In the ACC/AHA guidelines, aspirin, nitrates, and beta-blockers are recommended for all patients with ACS (MI and unstable angina) and are to be given immediately based on clinical history, even if the initial EKG is normal. Clopidogrel (Plavix) is recommended for all patients with ACS (non-ST MI, elevated MI, or unstable angina) who are not candidates for early angiography. In the wilderness setting, once the diagnosis of ACS is suspected, the patient should be treated aggressively with these four oral medications. The studies supporting these conclusions are:

1. ISIS-2 trial: Aspirin treatment reduced mortality by 23 percent in acute MI in prethrombolytic era (platelet cycloxygenase inhibitor).

2. Meta analysis of prethrombolytic era nitrate trials: Nitroglycerin treatment resulted in a 35 percent reduction in mortality from acute MI (vasodilator).

3. ISIS-I and MIAMI trials: Beta-blocker therapy resulted in 14 percent and 13 percent reduction in mortality with either atenolol or metoprolol in the prethrombolytic era (reduces heart rate, blood pressure, and ischemia; raises ventricular fibrillation threshold; and reduces likelihood of malignant ventricular arrhythmias and sudden death).

4. CURE trial: Clopidrogrel therapy resulted in an 18 percent reduction in MI, death, or stroke in patients with ACS and non-ST elevated MI treated medically (platelet ADP-receptor inhibitor).

II. ORAL MEDICATION PROTOCOL FOR PATIENTS WITH SUSPECTED ACUTE MYOCARDIAL INFARCTION OR UNSTABLE ANGINA PECTORIS (CATEGORY 1B)

A. Aspirin (81 mg, chewable)

Four tablets immediately, then one a day thereafter.

B. Nitroglycerin (0.4 mg tablets)

Dissolve sublingually every ten minutes, but do not give if BP is below 100 mmHg systolic. If no BP cuff is available, administer if the pulse is palpable in standing position and there are no signs of hypotension. Do not give if pulse is below 60/minute. Do not repeat if syncope develops after initial doses.

C. Clopidogrel

Give 300 mg (oral loading dose) immediately, then 75 mg a day. (Obese patients may require 600 mg loading dose for complete platelet inhibition.)

D. Beta-blockers

Administer metoprolol or atenolol (25 mg) every six hours, beginning thirty minutes after the onset of chest pain and repeated every six hours even if pain improves. Wait thirty minutes after onset of pain to identify patients with severe shock, bradycardia, or acute pulmonary edema. Do not give if heart rate is below 60/minute or BP is below 100 mmHg systolic or patient complains of severe shortness of breath or wheezing.

III. ADJUNCTIVE THERAPY FOR ACS PATIENTS IN THE WILDERNESS SETTING

A. Oxygen, if available, especially if at high altitude. Do not withhold oxygen because of concerns of limited oxygen supply ("what if we run out"): relieving ischemia may prevent the progression of acute LV dysfunction to fatal pulmonary edema.

B. Descent from high altitude (8,000 feet or 2,500 meters) is recommended if no supplemental oxygen is available.

C. Have patient assume semi-sitting position if possible. If shock develops, position head down and feet up to prevent downward spiral of BP and progressive coronary hypoperfusion.

D. Warm patient if cold.

E. If the victim is not in heart failure or shock, encourage fluid intake to avoid hypotension and dehydration.

F. Use nitrates for shortness of breath, just as you would for chest pain. Nitroglycerin will relieve pulmonary edema.

G. If evacuation is impossible (due to weather, terrain, third world location, ocean setting, etc.) and victim cannot self-rescue due to pain or shock, begin self-rescue to nearest hospital as soon as victim is able to move. Reinfarction is usually fatal. Continue aspirin, beta-blockers, and clopidogrel indefinitely until medical care is reached. Use nitrates as needed if exertional angina develops. Use nitroglycerin prophylactically during exertion every ten to fifteen minutes to prevent angina if self-rescue is attempted and efforts at self-rescue bring on chest pain.

H. Adjunctive pain medications with narcotics and antianxiety medications will help reduce ischemia and fear. Fifteen percent of patients are aspirin-resistant, and extra aspirin may help.

I. Pulmonary edema can be treated with rotating extremity tourniquets constructed of ACE bandages and rotated between limbs every ten minutes. Apply tourniquets enough to impede venous return, but not tight enough to cut off distal arterial pulsations.

J. Patients should be instructed early in the first minutes of their infarction to cough deeply and repetitively if they feel they are about to faint. Coughing will increase arterial pressure and prevent loss of consciousness during prolonged (minutes) of bradycardia or episodes of ventricular tachycardia.

Patients in ventricular fibrillation will lose consciousness immediately and will not be able to sustain consciousness for more than a few seconds despite coughing.

K. Brief episodes of unconsciousness and electromechanical collapse or cardiac arrest should be treated with CPR aggressively. Many inferior infarction patients will have two to three minutes of asystole, which will resolve with vigorous CPR and basic life support.

L. Sudden cardiac arrest should be treated with chest thumps in the hopes of converting a rapid V-tach to sinus rhythm.

M. Once cardiac arrest occurs, follow CPR guidelines for discontinuation if:
  1. Patient awakens
  2. Rescuers are exhausted
  3. Rescuers are in danger
  4. Patient is turned over to more definitive care
  5. Patient does not respond to prolonged (approximately thirty minutes) of resuscitative efforts

N. Continue to make efforts to seek hospitalization as soon as possible, even in remote third world settings, and arrange for assisted transport once a facility with defibrillator equipment is reached. Cardiac arrest may occur days or weeks after initial uneventful recovery of transmural MI.

IV. SPECIFIC SITUATIONS AND THE IMPLEMENTATION OF CPR

A. Hypothermia
Refer to chapter 11.

B. Avalanche victims
Breathless and pulseless victims of avalanches are usually dead from suffocation and/or blunt trauma. Hypothermia is often a compounding factor. Clear the airway, protect the cervical spine, and initiate rescue breathing and chest compressions (CPR) immediately.

Triage avalanche victims without vital signs at the scene according to the criteria of the ICAR Medical Commission (Category 1A):
  1. If there is no pulse and core temperature is 32°C or above, or burial is less than thirty minutes, continue CPR for twenty minutes. If successful with CPR, transfer to a hospital with an intensive care unit. If unsuccessful, stop CPR.

2. If the core temperature is below 32°C and burial is longer than thirty minutes, treatment depends upon the presence of an air pocket (any space around the nose or mouth, no matter how small).

a. If an air pocket is present, continue CPR and transfer to a hospital with cardiopulmonary bypass capability.

b. If no air pocket is present, stop CPR.

c. If an air pocket is possible, but not certain, continue and transfer to a hospital with cardiopulmonary bypass capability or to a closer hospital where potassium can be measured. Patients with serum potassium greater than 10 mmol/L have no chance of survival and are declared dead by asphyxiation. A field technique of rapid serum potassium determination will soon be available.

C. Cold-water submersion
Refer to chapter 3.

D. Lightning strike
Refer to chapter 14.

3

Submersion Injuries

Recommendations are considered Category 1B by the WMS Panel of Expert Reviewers.

I. GENERAL INFORMATION

Rescue of a near-drowning victim is inherently dangerous. The following guidelines are suggested for getting the victim safely out of the water:

- **Reach** for the victim, if possible, with an extended arm or leg, clothing, a stick or paddle, or anything that allows the rescuer to stay safely on land or in a boat.
- When reaching is not possible, **throw** something that floats to the victim.
- Throw a line to the victim and **tow** the victim to safety.
- **Row** or paddle out to drowning victims, in a boat, wearing a personal flotation device.
- Swimming rescues are extremely dangerous and are not recommended unless the rescuer has been trained and fully understands the risk involved. Do not attempt underwater searches for missing victims.

    All rescuers should wear personal flotation devices (PFDs).

II. GUIDELINES FOR ASSESSMENT AND TREATMENT

Assess unconscious patients immediately for adequate respiration. This can sometimes be done in the water, if the rescuer is a strong swimmer and/or if the rescuer can stand in shallow water. Begin rescue breathing as soon as possible. There is no value in attempting to clear the patient's lungs of water, but be prepared to roll the patient and clear the airway should water fill the airway during the rescue, or if the patient vomits. Dependent positioning to drain lungs of water is of no proven benefit. Protect the spine in unconscious patients and in the case of diving or surfing accidents. In the absence of a pulse, begin chest compressions as soon as possible. Continue CPR while pulseless, but terminate in thirty minutes if the pulse has not recovered. Evaluate all drowning and near-drowning patients for hypothermia. Hypothermic submersion patients cannot be presumed dead until they are "warm and dead." If they have been submersed for more than sixty minutes, or have not recovered a pulse after thirty minutes of CPR, they are dead.

Urgently evacuate all submersion patients to definitive medical care. Even if the victim feels "okay," it is possible to develop delayed respiratory, renal, or other problems, so evacuation is still indicated; the patient's vital signs should be monitored for twenty-four to forty-eight hours after submersion. Immediate treatment primarily by ventilation at the scene is the most important factor in determining survival. If the victim is unconscious or experiencing respiratory distress during transport, high-flow oxygen should be administered if available.

III. CONTROVERSIES

Should all victims of accidental submersion be evacuated?
Someone who is unexpectedly submersed and who comes up coughing but never loses consciousness does not need to be evacuated unless respiratory distress continues, or hypotension, bilateral crackles, and/or other signs of distress develop.

Should the Heimlich maneuver be used to clear the airway of a near-drowning victim?
The American Heart Association unequivocally recommends an immediate start of CPR without the Heimlich maneuver in the case of a near-drowned victim. Only utilize the Heimlich maneuver if foreign matter is suspected of obstructing the airway or when attempts to ventilate the patient fail due to a blocked airway.

CHAPTER

Traumatic Brain Injury

Recommendations are considered Category 1B by the WMS Panel of Expert Reviewers.

I. GENERAL INFORMATION

Anyone with a blow to the head or face, whether blunt or penetrating, risks developing increased intracranial pressure (ICP) or intracranial hemorrhage (ICH). Because definitive management of increasing ICP or ICH is not possible in the wilderness, prevention of head injuries should rank high among priorities. Prevention involves attention to safety and includes wearing an adequate helmet, approved for the specific activity being undertaken. It must fit the user and be held in place with a nonstretching chin strap. The use of even a properly fitted helmet does not preclude the possibility of a serious head injury, but it does reduce the risk. Chin straps should not obstruct venous blood flow as this may cause increased ICP.

II. GUIDELINES FOR ASSESSMENT

Some individuals after a blow to the head or face are low-risk and not in need of immediate evacuation. These patients have had relatively minor injuries. They do not lose consciousness or lose consciousness for only a brief period of time. They have no history of a bleeding disorder or the use of medications that might increase the risk of bleeding. Monitor patients in this category for twenty-four hours and awaken every two hours for assessment. Watch for:

- Alterations in mental status, including personality changes, lethargy, drowsiness, disorientation, unusual irritability, persistent retrograde amnesia, and combativeness
- Persistent nausea and vomiting
- Change in visual acuity
- Alterations in coordination and/or speech

If these signs or symptoms of increasing ICP appear, then an evacuation should be initiated.

Urgent evacuation is recommended for all patients who have received a blow to the head or face that results in loss of consciousness for more than a brief period of time or who have significant signs or symptoms of increasing ICP, or a depressed or basilar skull fracture. These signs and symptoms include:

- Debilitating headache
- Alterations in mental status (see above)
- Persistent nausea and vomiting
- Raccoon eyes (periorbital ecchymosis)
- Battle's sign (ecchymosis behind and below the ears)
- Loss of coordination
- Loss of visual acuity
- Appearance of clear fluid (possibly cerebral spinal fluid) from the nose and/or ears.
- Seizures
- Relapse into unconsciousness
- The inability to retain new memory

III. GUIDELINES FOR TREATMENT

If there is an obvious head injury, consider the possibility of a cervical spine injury (see chapter 5). Specific measures to implement during evacuation include the critical importance of establishing and maintaining an airway in all unconscious patients. Airway management, without specific adjuncts, can usually be accomplished by keeping the patient in a stable (preferably left-side) position, which also helps alleviate the possibility of aspirating vomitus, a common threat with head-injured patients. Alternatively, with consideration for possible spinal injury, place the patient with his/her entire body angled upward approximately 30 percent (reverse Trendelenburg position) to decrease the chance of aspiration and to decrease ICP. While all persons with a mechanism of injury that includes head involvement are strapped to a backboard in an urban setting, this is not necessary if the patient assessment does not indicate that evacuation is required. When evacuation is initiated, reassessment of the requirement for neck or spine immobilization should be made periodically. If the spine can be cleared, the rigid immobilization should be terminated, even through the evacuation process is continued.

IV. CONTROVERSIES

Does any loss of consciousness following a blow to the head warrant evacuation of the patient?

If the patient has been unconscious for only a brief period of time and/or with no obvious evidence of brain injury (see above), the patient may be left in the wilderness and carefully monitored for twenty-four hours.

What is meant by "a brief period of time" in relation to unconsciousness?

Seldom, if ever, is a period of unconsciousness accurately timed. The patient and/or witnesses are often unsure unconsciousness occurred. If a rescuer has been unable to get a response from a patient after aggressive stimulation, it may be assumed the patient has been unconscious for more than a brief period of time. Many authorities feel that a loss of consciousness for less than thirty seconds qualifies as a brief period of time, but consensus has not been reached on this topic.

5

Spinal Injury

Recommendations are considered Category 1B, except where indicated 1A, by the WMS Panel of Expert Reviewers.

I. GENERAL INFORMATION

In an urban environment, many patients placed in full spinal immobilization will prove to be free of unstable spine injuries. The inconvenience to patients and rescuers is worth the extra effort to protect the few with unstable spine injuries. In wilderness situations, spinal immobilization is difficult and can drastically alter the logistics of an evacuation. Immobilize all patients with signs or symptoms as indicated in the assessment section that follows. Patients with no signs or symptoms need not be immobilized despite significant mechanisms of injury, unless they have an altered level of responsiveness.

II. GUIDELINES FOR ASSESSMENT AND MANAGEMENT

In the wilderness a number of steps are involved in ruling out a spinal injury in a patient with a significant mechanism of injury. Treatment consists of full immobilization on a backboard or in a rigid litter, or immobilization on the most level ground available with a cervical collar until a rigid litter can be improvised or brought in. In the case of a patient with potential spinal injury whose ventilation is inadequate, the jaw thrust (rather than the head–tilt, chin lift) is the maneuver of choice to provide rescue breathing.

Before deciding to clear the spine, finish a full secondary assessment first to gain assurance the patient has no obvious signs and symptoms of spine injury and to assess the patient for distracting injuries. Distracting injuries are any conditions that cause pain or that might affect the patient's mental alertness. Conditions such as significant blood loss, alcohol use, fractures, or disturbed psychological status are a few examples. It is recommended that the rescuer perform a second and specific assessment relative to the spine before making the decision to clear the spine. The cervical spine can be clinically cleared if *all* of the following are met and documented (Category 1A) (reference: Hoffman, J. R., D. L. Schriger, W. Mower, et al. 1992. Low-risk criteria for cervical-spine radiography in blunt trauma: a prospective study. *Ann Emerg Med.* 21:1,454–60).

- The patient must be fully awake and alert, with no alcohol or medications that might alter his level of consciousness.
- The patient has no distracting injuries.
- The patient has a completely normal motor and sensory neurological examination.
- There is no pain or tenderness to palpation of the posterior cervical area, no palpable step-off deformity, and no other areas of pain to palpation over the thoracic or lumbar vertebra.

Spinal clearance is a continuous process. Reevaluation will be required, and the patient will have to be immobilized with cervical or full spinal splinting if any of the signs, symptoms, or conditions previously listed develop during the evacuation.

In the wilderness, full spinal immobilization may pose unnecessary hardship and danger to patients and rescuers. Therefore, seek a balance between the difficulties and dangers of evacuating an immobilized patient on one hand and not immobilizing a spinal injury on the other. In certain hazardous situations, it may be safer for the patient and rescuers to forego spinal immobilization, or to use only partial spinal immobilization, such as a cervical collar alone, to evacuate more easily and rapidly from the area of immediate danger.

6

Wound Management

Recommendations are considered Category 1B, except where indicated 1A or 2, by the WMS Panel of Expert Reviewers.

I. GENERAL INFORMATION

Assume contamination of open wounds and treat accordingly. The major goals are:

- Stop blood loss
- Clean the wound and keep it clean
- Promote healing and reduce discomfort
- Minimize loss of function

Most wilderness first-aid kits contain simple bandages and compresses only. Improvisation and the use of substitute materials are often required. Wilderness wounds are at risk for tetanus. Ensuring current tetanus immunization prior to participation in wilderness activities is encouraged.

II. GUIDELINES FOR ASSESSMENT AND TREATMENT

Wear fluid-barrier gloves when in contact with blood or other body fluids. Improvised personal protection could include, for example, a plastic food bag or a piece of garment to minimize contact with the victim's blood, and sunglasses or ski goggles to protect your eyes.

Even heavy bleeding can be controlled with pressure techniques in nearly all instances. Initially, apply direct digital pressure over the bleeding vessels and elevate the wound. Alternately, stop severe bleeding by placing two fingers, held together, into the wound. This temporary stasis is continued through the use of an internal pressure dressing made by taking a moist wad of gauze or clean cloth and packing it firmly into the wound. This is held in position with strips of gauze or tape.

These strips are not circumferentially tight but just cover and hold the packing gauze in place. Pressure points alone are not effective as a primary technique to control bleeding but may be useful as an adjunct. Arterial tourniquets are rarely necessary, but, if required to control bleeding, apply continuously until the patient reaches definitive surgical care (Category 1A). In a very remote area, where care might not be reached for days, continuous application will result in loss of the limb. Only in this situation will it be appropriate to release the tourniquet approximately every five minutes, *while continuing to apply direct wound pressure,* to assess the continued need for the tourniquet and to diminish the possibility of distal limb loss (Category 2). Assessment of continued bleeding can be accomplished within one second of release. Continuous tourniquet application is otherwise preferred to allowing additional heavy blood loss. (See the Controversies section that follows.)

A. Contusions

During the first forty-eight hours, contusions may be treated with cold compresses or cold-water immersion, and a compression dressing, to limit an expanding hematoma and to aid in pain relief. Apply cold for one half hour every two hours with due regard to possible cold injury. After seventy-two hours, apply heat in the same manner to promote healing. Topical heat ointments or creams can cause skin irritation, and their use is discouraged. Large contused areas with marked swelling cause severe pain and disability and may signal a large amount of blood loss or a significant underlying injury. Evaluate such patients for shock and other possible injuries and treat accordingly. Do not drain hematomas. A major soft tissue injury in proximity to a bone should arouse a high suspicion of a fracture. Apply splints for comfort.

B. Subungual hematomas

May be drained by drilling a hole in the nail with a red-hot paper clip, a sharp sterile blade, or hypodermic needle to provide pain relief.

C. Abrasions

May be cleaned with soap and water or with a surgical scrub such as 0.5 percent chlorhexidine gluconate or a 1 percent povidone-iodine impregnated sponge. Follow scrubbing with copious irrigation with clean water. Water safe to drink is clean enough for wound cleaning. After the abrasion has been cleaned, apply a thin coating of a topical antimicrobial first-aid ointment and dress with sterile gauze. If water is in short supply, the simple application of antibiotic ointment within three hours may reduce wound infection (Category 2). Honey and sugar are useful for field-expedient antisepsis.

D. Lacerations and avulsions

Use copious irrigation with clean water. Using water that is not at least potable is discouraged, unless the wound is grossly contaminated and no other irrigation is available. Boiled, then cooled, water is safest for open fractures or joints. Pressure irrigation with a syringe and needle or a barrel irrigation syringe is the most effective technique. Improvised equipment could include a plastic bag with a hole the size of a toothpick in it. Optimal pressure for irrigation is 5 to 8 psi, which would equal the force that could be applied to water using a barrel syringe with an 18 gauge needle. Irrigate with at least 500 ml of water. Take care to avoid splashing fluid into the irrigator's face. Following irrigation, inspect the wound and remove remaining debris with a sterile (flamed or boiled) forceps. If water is in limited supply, it may be helpful to irrigate grossly contaminated wounds with 1 percent povidone-iodine solution (not surgical scrub).

Do not close heavily contaminated or high-risk wounds because of the increased chance of wound infection. Pack heavily contaminated wounds open with wet-to-dry dressings. Wounds that open into joint spaces, that involve underlying tendons and ligaments, that open the face (for cosmetic reasons), that affect areas of special function (e.g., hands), and bites from wild animals (see chapter 19) are best cleaned and dressed without closure and the patient evacuated for definitive care. If evacuation is not feasible, or will take longer than two days, it is reasonable to treat significant wounds with thorough cleaning and closure with tape, wound-closure strips, sutures, or surgical staples. Minor wounds do not require urgent evacuation and may be closed with tape or wound-closure strips. Limit sharp debridement to obviously devitalized tissue. Splinting and elevation will help maintain wound closure, hemostasis, and pain control, although this is probably only feasible under limited circumstances.

If bone is exposed or if the wound is a deep puncture or highly contaminated, give appropriate antibiotics.

Traumatic amputations necessitate proper management of the amputated part if there will be any opportunity for reimplantation. Gently clean the amputated part and wrap in slightly moist sterile gauze, seal in plastic, and keep as cool as possible without freezing (ice water is best). Some parts, such as fingers, may be reattached up to thirty-two hours after the injury.

Ascertain tetanus status and give recommendations for updating after leaving the wilderness. Observe wounds daily for signs of infection that indicate the need for further irrigation, drainage, or debridement.

III. GUIDELINES FOR EVACUATION

Rapid evacuation from the wilderness is advisable for:

- Severe animal bites or bites from potentially rabid animals
- Deep or highly contaminated wounds with a high risk of infection
- Infected wounds not responding to reasonable field treatment
- Wounds associated with severe blood loss.

While not urgent, consider evacuation for wounds that severely limit a person's ability to participate in the trip and wounds that require closure for cosmetic reasons (such as facial wounds). Delayed primary closure of facial wounds can be performed in three to five days if the wound is kept clean with daily packing.

IV. CONTROVERSIES

Should wounds be closed in the wilderness?

Although sterile techniques are virtually impossible in the wilderness, primary closure with sutures, staples, or wound-closure strips may be feasible for relatively clean wounds. Staples provide a cosmetic result identical to that of interrupted sutures, but not subcuticular sutures. The patient's comfort and ability and willingness to function are increased, and healing time is usually shortened. For ulcerations, abscess cavities, deep puncture wounds, and animal bites, do not close wounds but allow to gradually heal by granulation and eventual reepithelization. Grossly contaminated wounds, such as those excessively contaminated with soil or feces, must be cleaned and observed for four to five days before closure, if the wilderness trip lasts that long.

Should antibiotic prophylaxis be considered for wilderness wounds?

The following are general indications for antibiotic prophylaxis:

- Significantly contaminated wounds requiring extensive cleaning and debridement (especially in patients with preexisting valvular heart disease, prosthetic joints, or immunosuppressed patients)
- Violation of cartilage, joint spaces, tendon, or bone
- Crush-mechanism wounds with a high potential for devitalization
- Mammalian bites (see chapter 19)

For prophylaxis use amoxicillin-clavulanate, a second- or third-generation cephalosporin, a quinolone, a penicillinase-resistant penicillin, or a tetracycline antibiotic. Five days of prophylactic therapy suffice.

Should tourniquets be released every five minutes with continued direct pressure to assess clotting, or should tourniquets be left in place once applied until definitive medical care has been reached?

Several military studies have indicated an increased death rate if tourniquets are removed, even temporarily, in the field. The reason for reassessing clotting with direct pressure and attempting tourniquet release has been that wilderness evacuations might take days or even weeks to accomplish. A tourniquet used for that length of time would result in necrosis of the distal limb with devastating consequences for the injured patient. Additionally, arterial tourniquets are extremely painful in a conscious individual. In the wilderness the patient would receive constant care, not intermittent care as may be the case in battlefield circumstances, but it is essential to not allow additional blood loss with sequential removals of the tourniquet.

7

Burn Management

Recommendations are considered Category 1B, except where indicated 1A, by the WMS Panel of Expert Reviewers.

I. GENERAL INFORMATION

The most likely source of major burn trauma in the outdoors is from scalds from hot liquids. Thermal injuries from stoves, carbide lights and lanterns, hot utensils, and campfires are generally not extensive. Burns from UV exposure are possible during cloudy days. UV is more intense at high altitudes and low latitudes and can be enhanced by reflection from snow, water, and sand.

II. GUIDELINES FOR ASSESSMENT AND TREATMENT

Every aspect of burn treatment depends on assessment of the depth and extent of the injury. Although this assessment may be an estimate, it is the basis for deciding how the patient will be treated, and whether evacuation is required and how urgently.

A. Assessment

1. Depth

Superficial burns involve the epidermis only. The skin color is red to pale, and no blister forms. Partial thickness burns have blisters in addition to the red discoloration of the skin. Full thickness burns have a pale or charred skin color and do not have blister formation. The initial level of pain in a burned area can give a clue as to how deep the burn is. Partial thickness burns are frequently very painful; deep partial thickness burns can have little pain but still have pressure sensation. Full thickness burns are painless and have no pressure sensation (skin nerves are destroyed).

2. Extent

Use the Rule of Nines, in which each arm represents approximately 9 percent of a person's total body surface area (TBSA), each leg 18 percent (the front of the leg 9 percent, and the back of the leg 9 percent), the front of the torso 18 percent, the back of the trunk 18 percent, the head 9 percent, and the groin 1 percent. For infants and small children, the head represents a larger percentage (18 percent) and the legs a smaller percentage (13.5 percent). For smaller areas use the Rule of Palmar Surface: The patient's entire palmar surface (the surface of palm and fingers) equals about 1 percent TBSA. Only count partial thickness and full thickness burns in the estimate of total body surface area burned.

3. Pain

In addition to depth and extent, also include an assessment of pain. Adequate control of pain is a treatment goal and indicator of the ability to manage a burn wound while in the wilderness. If you cannot manage the pain, your treatment is inadequate.

4. Location

Burns to the face, genitals, palms, or soles require evacuation.

B. Initial care

1. Stop the burning process. The faster the better, within thirty seconds if possible. Heat can continue to injure tissue as long as a material with a temperature above 65°C is in contact with the skin. No first aid will be effective until the burning process has stopped. Smother flames, if appropriate, and then cool the burn with water with due regard to causing hypothermia in an extensively burned patient. Remove clothing and all jewelry, especially rings or other constricting items. Remove rings even if the hands are not burned. Do not try to remove anything that has stuck to the wound.

2. Manage airway, breathing, and circulation (the ABCs) with particular attention to the possibility of thermal injury to the airway. Signs and symptoms of thermal airway injury include:

- Hoarse or muffled voice
- Soot in mouth
- Carbonaceous sputum
- Singed nasal hair
- Significant burns to the face

If there is any suspicion of airway injury, early definitive management of the airway is needed and emergency evacuation should be initiated. Administer oxygen to all suspected airway-burn victims, those with smoke inhalation, and to all others with critical burns.

3. Assess for associated injuries such as fractures or lacerations and inhalation injury.

4. Evaluate the burn (depth, extent, pain, and location).

5. General treatment for the patient.

    a. Stabilize the body temperature. When skin is lost, so is the patient's ability to thermoregulate and prevent heat loss.

    b. Elevate injured parts.

    c. Hydration is of critical importance in long-term care. Have the patient drink as much fluid as he/she can tolerate, unless the patient complains of nausea. Avoid vomiting, if possible. Include some salt in the oral fluids, but do not make these solutions stronger than 0.9 percent.

    d. Remember: In the early stages of burn injury, altered consciousness is due to a cause other than the burn.

C. General treatment of the burn

Caring for the wound itself is often the least important aspect of burn care. All burn wounds are sterile for the first twenty-four to forty-eight hours. Burn management is aimed primarily at keeping the wound clean, reducing the pain, and regulating fluid status and body temperature.

    1. Gently wash the burn with slightly warm water and mild soap, if needed, to remove any debris and to clean the skin surface around the burn site. Pat dry. Remove the skin from blisters that have popped open or are hemorrhagic (but do not open blisters).

    2. Cover the patient with a dry sterile dressing and do not use topical antibiotic ointments if the patient can get to a burn unit within twenty-four hours. Otherwise, dress burns with a thin layer of antibiotic ointment.

    3. Cover the burn with a gel dressing if the burn is small enough, or cover with a thin layer of gauze, or with clean, dry clothing. Covering wounds reduces pain and evaporative losses. Superficial burns can benefit from inexpensive moisturizing cream or aloe vera creams. The use of hyperosmolar solutions such as honey or sugar is acceptable as a field expedient dressing.

    4. When evacuation is imminent, do not re-dress or reexamine the injury. If evacuation is prolonged, re-dress once daily. Remove old dressings, reclean (removing the old ointment), and apply fresh ointment and a clean dry covering. (*NOTE:* Soak off old dressings with clean, tepid water.)

    5. Do not pack wounds in ice. Start cooling within thirty minutes of the injury, but do not continue for longer than thirty minutes. If the burn is 9 percent TBSA or less, the cooling can be applied for longer than thirty minutes if needed for pain control (Category 1A) (reference: Marx, J. A., R. S. Hockberger, MD, and R. M. Walls, MD. 2002. *Rosen's emergency medicine, concepts and clinical practice.* 5th ed. p. 807. St. Louis, Mo.: Mosby).

6. Elevate burned extremities to minimize swelling. Swelling retards healing and encourages infection. Have the patient gently and regularly move burned areas as much as possible.

7. Ibuprofen is probably the best oral over-the-counter analgesic for burn pain (including sunburn).

8. If you have no ointment or dressings, leave the burn alone. The burn's surface will dry into a scablike covering that provides protection.

III. GUIDELINES FOR EVACUATION

Superficial burns, even extensive ones, rarely require evacuation. Although they do not require urgent evacuation, blistered burns greater than 1 percent TBSA are difficult to keep clean in the wilderness and should be evacuated. Partial thickness burns covering less than 15 percent TBSA must receive definitive care but seldom warrant urgent evacuation. Full thickness burns need definitive medical care to heal best but do not usually require urgent evacuation unless they are extensive. Partial thickness and full thickness burns covering more than 15 percent TBSA are often a threat to life, requiring urgent evacuation. Any serious burn to the face or above the nipple line may have burned the patient's airway and must be considered an urgent evacuation. Urgently evacuate patients with deep burns to hands, feet, genitals, eyes, or mucous membranes, or circumferential burns. Urgently evacuate chemical and electrical burns.

8

Orthopedic Injuries

Recommendations are considered Category 1B, unless where indicated 1A, by the WMS Panel of Expert Reviewers.

I. GENERAL INFORMATION

Sprains, strains, and fractures, especially injuries to lower extremities, are among the most common accidents in wilderness settings. The treatment of these injuries may vary, depending upon the expertise and experience of those in the party and the distance from definitive medical help. In remote settings, making the patient as functional as possible is often the overriding concern, thereby facilitating self-rescue and eliminating the need for outside assistance. Remember, the safety of the group takes precedence over optimal treatment of any individual injury.

Managing fractures in remote environments requires common sense, good diagnostic skills, and sensitivity to the needs of the patient and the group. For example, in a severe ankle injury where a fracture is suspected, one would normally immobilize the part and put the patient on crutches with instructions for elevation, ice, and rest from weight-bearing. In the wilderness, however, one must weigh other factors: the desire of the patient to ambulate on a suspicious ankle injury, the availability of people to transport the patient, the type of terrain involved in transport, the severity of the environment, distance involved, and the patient's need or desire as well as ability to continue carrying a load. Thus, whereas the best medical judgment precludes weight-bearing, the best decision in a remote environment might be to immobilize the ankle in a splint, or tape the ankle securely as for an athletic event, and allow the patient to hobble along on his or her good ankle, using an ice axe, ski pole, or wooden stick for balance. This could be the safest and most reasonable decision based on the situation.

II. GUIDELINES FOR ASSESSMENT AND TREATMENT

A. Fractures

In the wilderness, without a radiographic picture of the involved bones, assessment of a fracture includes the following questions:

- Are there obvious signs of a fracture, such as angulations, swelling, or bruising?
- Can the patient move the injury, or does she/he guard it carefully?
- Is there crepitation with movement?
- Is there point tenderness with palpation of the site, or pain at the suspected injury site with axial compression along the long bone or with torque on the bone?
- Is there discoloration and swelling?
- How does the injured side compare to the uninjured side?
- Does the injury feel rigid, with spasm of the surrounding muscles?
- Did the patient feel or hear anything break?
- What was the mechanism of injury? (High-speed impacts cause more fractures than low-speed impacts.)
- Is there adequate circulation distal to the suspected fracture site?
- How willing is the patient to use the injured area? Is the patient able to bear any weight or load on the affected limb?

The key elements of a splint are adequate padding for comfort and adequate rigidity for safety without compromise of distal circulation. Splinting may be accomplished with formal splints or improvised splints, e.g., clothing, adhesive or athletic tape, foam sleeping pads, ice axes, ski poles, or natural material. The patient is the best source of information on how well splints are working. Peripheral pulses or capillary refill, as well as neurologic function distal to the injury, must be monitored before and after all splinting. Recheck pulses, capillary refill, distal limb color, and nerve function (sensation and movement) periodically to ensure that the splint wrap is not too tight. It is important to give the patient the responsibility of notifying someone of any changes in sensation or level of pain.

1. Shoulder

Fractures of the shoulder girdle are quite often stable and require nothing more than sling immobilization, cold compresses (if available), and allowance for gentle motion of the forearm and hand. A fracture of the clavicle may be treated with a sling and swathe. The hand and wrist must be accessible for feeling pulses.

2. Upper arm

The humeral shaft is palpable on the medial side throughout its entire length. Therefore, when a fracture is suspected, palpate the length of the humerus, beginning either proximal or distal to the patient's area of complaint. In this way, very small, nondisplaced fractures may be identified. Ask the patient to extend her or his wrist, digits, and thumb to check the radial nerve function and document for future reference. Immobilizing the arm against the body wall is nature's best splint. Humeral fractures can be very adequately padded and immobilized in this manner with a sling and swathe. For comfort leave the elbow free and dependent, allowing gravity to apply gentle traction to the fracture site, which is splinted to the thorax with only the swathe. An unstable or displaced humeral fracture may require a padded splint.

3. Lower arm

Adequately splint fractures of the elbow, forearm, and wrist, incorporating the joints above and below. If possible, splint the elbow at eighty to ninety degrees of flexion to elevate the forearm and hand and reduce swelling.

The stability provided by a rigid splint is worth the effort, especially in a long and difficult transport. Splint fractures of the distal ulna and radius with the hand placed in the position of function with a rolled-up sock, glove, or other soft material tucked into the palm. Then immobilize the hand, wrist, and forearm in a splint. Active exercise of the hand is quite helpful in promoting circulation.

Correct marked angulation. Applying a splint to a badly angulated forearm fracture is difficult and usually unstable. Gentle traction with an assistant applying counter-traction to the upper arm results in an overall improvement, with a negligible risk of creating further vascular or neurologic damage. Move slowly and stop if force is required for further movement, or if the patient complains of significantly increasing pain.

4. Hand

Fractures of the hand are often associated with dislocations of the proximal or distal interphalangeal joints. Reduce phalangeal fractures and splint in a position of function as indicated above, not in an extended position. Immediately after injury, these fractures can be reduced with only minimal discomfort. Hours after the injury, swelling and pain make realignment more difficult. Use of an ice compress and very gentle traction can realign fractures of the hand without significant discomfort. Immobilize the digits in a position of function whenever possible, and use adjacent digits for splinting (the "buddy system"). Place gauze between the buddy-taped fingers to absorb moisture and prevent skin ulceration. A suitable hand splint may be made by placing the entire hand in a functional position with a soft roll of material in the palm, and then wrapping the whole with an elastic wrap or roller gauze. Torn strips of clothing can be used for an improvised hand splint.

5. Hip

In fractures of the hip, the typical position of external rotation and shortening of the leg may or may not be present. The fracture may be an impacted femoral neck type or an acetabular fracture. Diagnosis might be difficult. As a general guideline, if a patient has sustained significant trauma and has very painful motion in the region of the hip, plus pain with weight-bearing, carry him or her out on a litter or sled. Do not place suspected fractures of the hip in traction. Secure the leg on the affected side to the uninjured leg for splinting.

6. Pelvis

In suspected fractures of the pelvis, treat for shock due to the massive blood loss often associated with this injury. Because of possible bladder trauma, check for hematuria. Gentle constricting wraps placed around the pelvic region may provide temporary comfort and more stability to the fracture. A Therm-a-Rest pad, secured around the pelvis and then inflated, offers excellent improvised pelvic stability. The patient requires stabilization on a rigid backboard, litter, or sled and urgent evacuation.

7. Femur

While pain is relieved with initial manual traction, placing a person in a traction splint is technically difficult and can result in complications from tissue necrosis due to pressure points, compromised circulation, and complications of extraction due to the length of the traction device. Closely observing the compression of the traction system is mandatory and causes heat loss during cold weather, due to the temporary opening of the thermal wrap.

A traction splint is no more efficacious than a good packaging technique. Immobilize the fractured extremity to the uninjured leg with adequate padding. When long transport is anticipated, place padding behind the knee to create 5 to 10 percent knee flexion. This position is much more comfortable than if the knee is fully extended.

8. Knee

Patellar fractures from a fall directly on the knee may be difficult to differentiate from a severe contusion unless there is an obvious deformity. A person with a comminuted fracture of the patella will be unable to extend the knee. Immobilize a patient with severe knee pain in a cylinder splint that stabilizes the knee and allows the patient to walk with assistance. Improvise a cane or crutch if terrain and other factors dictate that this is the best course of action.

9. Lower leg

Splint tibia and both bone fractures to incorporate the knee and ankle. Many isolated fibula fractures require only an ankle splint, and the victim can ambulate with a cane or crutch. Traction splinting is unnecessary. Gently correct angular deformities (see "lower arm").

10. Ankle

Fractures of the ankle may be difficult to assess. The Ottowa Ankle Rules indicate a fracture might exist (literally that an X-ray is indicated) if there is tenderness over the inferior or posterior pole of either malleolus, including the distal malleolus (Category 1A) (reference: Dunlop, M. G., T. F. Beattie, G. K. White, G. M. Raab, and R. I. Doull. 1986. Guidelines for selective radiographic assessment of inversion ankle injuries. *BMJ* [Clin Res Ed] 293:603–5). Early examination and treatment are important. Immobilize adequately, then elevate and apply cold to the injured extremity. A well-wrapped compression dressing is also quite helpful. Ankle fractures may be splinted very well with parkas, foam sleeping pads, or other comparable gear arranged in a U shape around the foot and lower leg.

11. Foot

Specific indications of a midfoot fracture are tenderness along the base of the fifth metatarsal or navicular bone and the inability to bear weight (four steps) at the time of the injury and at the time of examination (Category 1A) (reference as indicated under "ankle"). Splinting is similar as for ankle fractures. Ambulation may be possible for self-evacuation, especially when aided by a cane or crutch.

B. Dislocations

It is important to diagnose and reduce a dislocation quickly after it occurs. Discretion must obviously be used in deciding to reduce the dislocation when evacuation to a nearby medical facility can be easily accomplished. Always examine and document motor, sensory, and circulatory status distal to the dislocation both before and after attempted reductions.

The major advantages of early reduction are:

- Reduction is easier immediately after the injury, before swelling and muscle spasm have developed.
- Transport of the patient is easier after reduction.
- Reduction usually results in dramatic relief of pain.
- Immobilization of the injured joint is easier to accomplish and more stable after reduction.
- The safety of the entire party may be jeopardized during the evacuation of a patient with a major joint dislocation.
- Early reduction reduces the circulatory and neurological risks to the extremity.

Signs helpful in identifying a dislocation include:

- Restriction of motion through the joint's normal range
- Obvious deformity in comparison with the uninvolved side

- Crepitus or grating of bone fragments is absent
- Often a typical, identifiable posture of the dislocated joint, which the patient will maintain to minimize pain

Obtaining a history of the mechanism of injury is helpful.

Avulsion fractures may accompany dislocations. The alignment of these fractures is usually improved with the reduction of the dislocation. The same is true of vessel or nerve impairment associated with a dislocation. When a major long bone fracture (e.g., femur or humerus) accompanies a dislocation in the same area, the dislocation may not even be diagnosed in view of the more apparent major fracture. In these cases, splinting of the fracture is the main concern. The dislocation, for all practical purposes, is a secondary issue and usually not amenable to reduction by ordinary means.

1. Shoulder

Anterior-inferior dislocations of the shoulder joint account for more than 95 percent of shoulder dislocations. The mechanism of injury is usually external rotation and abduction. The problem is often recurrent, and the patient can identify the dislocation quite readily. The patient will usually stabilize the shoulder in the most comfortable position but cannot bring the involved extremity across the chest to a position of rest. The upper arm is held away from the body in various positions and cannot be brought into a sling-type position. This differentiates a dislocation from a fracture of the humerus, in which the patient usually splints the upper arm against the chest wall for comfort. Check circulation, motor and sensory function to the hand, and also sensory function along the outer aspect of the shoulder (axillary nerve), and document findings.

Posterior dislocations of the shoulder are not common and tend to occur mainly with electrical injuries or tonic-clonic seizures. In this instance, the upper arm and forearm are held across the anterior chest wall, and attempts at externally rotating the upper arm away from the chest are restricted and painful. The diagnosis is often difficult to make.

One method for reduction of an anterior shoulder dislocation is steady traction with the arm abducted ninety degrees, pulling straight from the body with counter-traction provided in the region of the axilla by an assistant. Muscle relaxation through massage can enhance attempts at relocation and is appropriate. Be sure to pad the axilla and the antecubital region to protect nerve and vascular structures during traction.

A second method is to place the patient prone and let the arm hang down toward the ground with ten to fifteen pounds of weight secured to the hand. This method may be slow, and relaxation is critically important, but the muscles will generally fatigue in time, and manual assistance by manipulation of the shoulder is helpful.

After reduction, immobilize the shoulder with sling and swathe.

2. Elbow

Look for obvious deformity when compared to the uninvolved side and restricted flexion and extension of the joint. Most commonly, the olecranon dislocates toward the rear, and a bony prominence shows posteriorly.

Apply slow, steady traction to the forearm in a partially flexed position with counter-traction applied to the upper arm by an assistant. The patient's ability to fully flex the elbow is a sign of reduction. The joint may be displaced medially or laterally and may require side pressure for realignment. After reduction, immobilize in a sling and swathe. If reduction is not possible, splint in the position found.

3. Wrist

Wrist dislocations are very difficult to differentiate from a fracture and often are difficult to reduce. Splint immobilization is the treatment of choice (see "lower arm" in the Fractures section). Circulation and neurologic function to the hand are usually not compromised, but if they are, attempt reduction with gentle in-line traction.

4. Fingers

Obvious deformity and limited function are the main diagnostic factors. Reduction of dislocations of middle and distal interphalangeal joints is accomplished by maintaining the digit in partial flexion and pushing the dislocated base of the phalanx back in place while traction is applied to the partially flexed digit.

There are two hand dislocations in which reduction is difficult, if not impossible, by closed means: dislocation of the metacarpophalangeal joint of the index finger and the metacarpophalangeal joint of the thumb. The thumb is sometimes reducible closed, but the index metacarpal rarely is. Make one attempt, and then immobilize the joint in a functional position. Do not persist with multiple attempts.

5. Hip

The majority of dislocations are posterior. The hip will be moderately flexed, internally rotated, and adducted. Any attempt to extend the hip for splinting or easier transport will be resisted by the patient and is mechanically nearly impossible to accomplish. Anterior dislocation of the hip results in a posture of extension, external rotation, and adduction. Again, attempting to extend the hip to a neutral position is very difficult, if not impossible, and is resisted by the patient.

If skill and equipment are available, the use of intramuscular or intravenous muscle relaxants or analgesics greatly facilitate any reduction. This reduction requires two people, ideally, with one applying counter-traction to the pelvis with the patient lying in a supine position on the ground. In the case of a posterior hip dislocation, the involved hip and knee are flexed to ninety degrees, with the rescuer straddling the patient and applying traction in an upward direction. If only one person is available to attempt the reduction, the victim can be placed prone over a log, rock, or bench, and the traction applied downward with hip and knee flexed ninety degrees. Once reduced, the injured hip must be immobilized to the uninvolved extremity, and the patient must be transported in a supine position.

6. Patella

Most often, the patella is laterally displaced, with the knee held in flexion for comfort. Such an injury is often recurrent and caused by a pivoting type of injury with a partially flexed knee. The patella is not movable and is obviously out of place.

Flex the hip to relax the quadriceps, and then apply gentle traction to extend the knee. In most cases, the patella will slip back into its groove. Applying direct, gentle pressure to the patella from the lateral aspect may be necessary to attain reduction. Immobilize the extremity with a cylinder splint. With the knee extended and immobilized, the patient may be able to walk well enough for self-evacuation.

7. Knee

Major ligamentous disruption is the rule in dislocations of the knee. The knee may not be dislocated at the time of exam, but gross instability is the major clue, and vascular impairment is an important risk. Check pulses and motor function in ankle and foot.

Gentle realignment of the joint benefits damaged neurovascular structures. Splint securely, without compromising circulation to the foot. The patient must be carried out.

8. Ankle

Most commonly associated with fractures, the dislocated ankle is obviously deformed and often manifests crepitus. Reduce the deformity as much as possible as necrosis of tight, stretched overlying skin is a danger. Ordinarily, this is not difficult because of the gross instability resulting from associated fractures. Hold the forefoot, and allow the remainder of the extremity to act as the counter-traction. Improved alignment of the ankle dislocation results without much additional effort. Gentle traction of the heel and foot also helps. Immobilize with a splint, and carry the patient out.

III. GUIDELINES FOR EVACUATION

Deciding which injuries mandate premature termination of a trip, and how rapidly and by what means evacuation will be performed, is a function of both the type of trip and type of injury. Urgent evacuation is indicated in:

■ Open fractures
■ Injuries with vascular compromise not alleviated by reduction

- Spinal injuries with neurologic deficits
- Injuries associated with significant blood loss, major fractures (hip, femur, pelvis, injury with deformity at the knee, ankle, or elbow)
- Major dislocation that cannot be reduced
    Evacuation is not needed for:
- Digit injuries
- Minimal injuries to other joints

With adequate splinting, delays in reaching definitive medical care often result in no permanent harm.

9

Eye Pathology

Recommendations are considered Category 1B by the WMS Panel of Expert Reviewers.

I. GENERAL INFORMATION

Management of ocular emergencies in the wilderness is made more difficult by three factors: the lack of diagnostic equipment, such as a slit lamp; the lack of specialty consultation; and limited medications with which to treat the disorders encountered. Typical of many wilderness medical management issues, the diagnostic and therapeutic approaches presented in this chapter are not necessarily to be used when professional referral is readily available.

This guideline discusses sudden vision loss in a noninflamed eye, orbital and periorbital inflammation, and the acute red eye. The available medications and equipment with which to treat these disorders will be assumed to be those in the recommended wilderness ocular emergency kit that follows.

II. MEDICATIONS AND EQUIPMENT

The proposed management of ocular emergencies in the wilderness requires that the following medications and equipment are available to the treating medical personnel.

WILDERNESS EYE KIT MEDICATIONS

- Gatifloxacin 0.3 percent drops or moxifloxacin 0.5 percent drops
- Tetracaine 0.5 percent drops
- Prednisolone acetate 1 percent drops
- Gatifloxacin or moxifloxacin 400 mg tabs
- Bacitracin ophthalmic ointment
- Prednisone 20 mg tabs
- Artificial tears
- Scopolamine 0.25 percent drops
- Diclofenac 0.1 percent drops
- Pilocarpine 2 percent drops

WILDERNESS EYE KIT EQUIPMENT	
■ Penlight with cobalt blue filter	■ Eye patches (or equal)
■ Fluorescein strips	■ 1-inch tape
■ Cotton-tipped applicators	■ Wound-closure strips ($\frac{1}{4}$ inch, or make
■ Metal eye shield (or rig from suitable	from wider tape)
material)	■ Magnifying glass

III. GUIDELINES FOR ASSESSMENT AND TREATMENT

When confronted by ocular disorders in the wilderness, attempt to measure the visual acuity. Reading the print in a book or any other printed material will provide at least a rough measure of visual acuity.

A. Acute vision loss in the noninflamed eye

Disorders that may cause acute visual loss in a noninflamed eye include retinal detachment, central retinal artery occlusion, anterior ischemic optic neuropathy, optic neuritis, central retinal vein occlusion, arteritic anterior ischemic optic neuropathy, vitreous hemorrhage, and significant high-altitude retinal hemorrhage. These disorders are difficult to diagnose and treat in the wilderness, and, in most cases, all that can be done is to arrange for an urgent evacuation.

1. Giant Cell Arteritis (GCA)

A key question that must be asked is, "Does the patient have Giant Cell Arteritis?" This is important because visual loss in one eye due to GCA is often rapidly followed by visual loss in the other eye if untreated. In addition, untreated GCA has a significant mortality. Diagnostic factors that may help to identify a person with GCA are age greater than fifty-five, temporal headache, jaw claudication, fever, weight loss, previous transient episodes of visual loss, and generalized muscle aches and fatigue. If GCA is suspected, start the individual on 80 mg a day of prednisone and evacuate on an urgent basis.

2. Central retinal artery occlusion

The other cause of acute visual loss in a noninflamed eye that may sometimes be treated successfully in the wilderness is central retinal artery occlusion. For this reason, treat acute loss of vision in the wilderness with a trial of supplemental oxygen, if available, at the highest inspired fraction achievable as soon as possible after the onset of symptoms. If supplemental oxygen is to be of any benefit, a response is typically seen within just a few minutes.

B. Orbital or periorbital inflammation

This may result from preseptal cellulitis, orbital cellulitis, orbital pseudotu-mor, insect envenomation, or dacryocystitis. Preseptal cellulitis is character-ized by periocular erythema and edema, a history of periocular trauma or hordeolum, no proptosis, no restriction of extraocular motility, no diplopia, and no change in visual acuity. Treatment for preseptal cellulitis is gatifloxacin or moxifloxacin (400 mg, once a day), with expedited evacuation if no improve-ment is seen in twenty-four to forty-eight hours. Dacryocystitis is a specific type of preseptal cellulitis in which the source of the infection is an obstructed nasolacrimal duct. The erythema and inflammation are localized to the area overlying the lacrimal sac at the inferior nasal aspect of the lower eyelid. It is treated in the same manner as previously described, except that warm com-presses should also be used. The diagnosis of periocular insect envenomation is made when the periocular erythema and edema are associated with an insect envenomation by history or by identification of a papular or vesicular lesion at the site of envenomation. Treatment is with cool compresses and antihista-mines. Also give gatifloxacin or moxifloxacin (400 mg, once a day) if second-ary infection is suspected on the basis of increasing pain, redness, or swelling. Orbital cellulitis will also have periocular erythema and edema, but these signs will typically be accompanied by a history of sinusitis or upper respira-tory tract infection, proptosis, diplopia, restricted extraocular motility, decreased visual acuity, and/or fever. Orbital cellulitis is a life-threatening disorder and is treated with gatifloxacin or moxifloxacin (400 mg, once a day), deconges-tants, and urgent evacuation.

C. Acute red eye

The differential diagnosis of the acute red eye includes both obvious and occult open globe injury, corneal abrasion or ulcer, subconjunctival hemorrhage, trau-matic and nontraumatic iritis, hyphema, herpes simplex virus keratitis, corneal erosion, acute angle-closure glaucoma, scleritis, conjunctivitis, blepharitis, ultra-violet keratitis, episcleritis, conjunctival foreign body, dry eye, and contact lens overwear syndrome. There a few simple diagnostic steps that can be under-taken that will help to differentiate between the entities listed.

DIAGNOSTIC APPROACH TO ACUTE RED EYE IN THE WILDERNESS	
Trauma	**No Trauma**
■ Obvious open globe	■ Fluorescein test
■ Fluorescein test	■ Response to topical anesthesia
	■ Pupillary status

The first step is to inquire whether there has been recent trauma to the eye. If there has, the eye should be checked with a light source immediately to see if there is an obvious open globe. This type of injury is most often encountered in the presence of lacerating or impaling trauma, such as from a knife wound, a fishhook, or a tree branch or thorn impaling the globe. Should an obvious open globe be noted, immediately place a rigid shield (not a pressure patch) over the eye to protect it from further trauma. Start the victim immediately on gatifloxacin or moxifloxacin (400 mg, once daily) and arrange for an urgent evacuation. Posttraumatic infection of the eye (called endophthalmitis) is a dreaded complication of an open globe and often results in permanent loss of vision.

If there is a history of eye trauma but no obvious open globe, perform a fluorescein stain with a fluorescein strip and a drop of topical anesthesia. If an epithelial defect is seen with the cobalt blue light, the victim has either a corneal abrasion or a corneal ulcer. Several factors will help to differentiate the two. A corneal ulcer will often be seen as a white or gray spot on the cornea with a tangential penlight examination. No opacities or infiltrates are seen with a corneal abrasion. In addition, a corneal ulcer typically takes a day or two to develop after an episode of trauma and may be accompanied by a discharge. Increasing pain and photophobia are usually present with a developing corneal ulcer.

A traumatic corneal abrasion is treated with gatifloxacin 0.3 percent drops or moxifloxacin 0.5 percent drops four times a day to prevent infection. Diclofenac 0.1 percent drops four times a day may be added for pain control. (Wait five minutes between drops.) Sunglasses are helpful in reducing irritation from light if the eye is not patched. Patching of abrasions is no longer routinely done, but it is an option for very large abrasions or if the individual gets significant pain relief from the patch. If the eye is patched because of a large or very painful abrasion, use bacitracin ointment before patching and recheck the eye in twenty-four hours. Depth perception will be affected by patching, so the individual will need to use care to not incur a secondary injury from a fall if he or she is moving across the terrain in a wilderness setting. Scopolamine 0.25 percent, one drop bid or before patching, may be added for very painful abrasions, but it will result in blurring of near vision and a dilated pupil for three to six days. Systemic analgesics may also be required in some cases. Remove the patch daily to check for the development of a corneal ulcer and to repeat the fluorescein stain to monitor healing. Healing of the abrasion should occur within one to three days. If the trauma causing the abrasion is related to contact lens wear or insertion, there is a higher incidence of secondary infection with gram negative organisms, and the eye should *not* be patched. Use gatifloxacin 0.3 percent drops or moxifloxacin 0.5 percent drops every two hours while awake until the abrasion is healed, and watch the eye closely for development of a corneal ulcer.

If the diagnosis of corneal ulcer is made on the basis of trauma, an epithelial defect, and a white or gray spot on the cornea, treat with gatifloxacin 0.3 percent drops or moxifloxacin 0.5 percent drops as follows: one drop every five minutes for five doses; one drop every thirty minutes for six hours; then one drop every hour around the clock. Scopolamine 0.25 percent may be added for pain control if needed. A corneal ulcer is a vision-threatening disorder that may progress rapidly despite therapy, so an expedited evacuation should be arranged. A posttraumatic red eye without an obvious open globe or an epithelial defect on fluorescein staining may represent a subconjunctival hemorrhage, traumatic iritis, hyphema, or an occult ruptured globe. A subconjunctival hemorrhage is a bright red area of blood overlying the sclera of the eye. It requires no treatment, but a careful inspection of the eye for associated injuries should be made. If the subconjunctival hemorrhage is massive and causes outward bulging of the conjunctiva (called chemosis), then suspect an occult ruptured globe and manage as previously described for an obvious open globe.

Blood in the anterior chamber of the eye is called a hyphema. The primary concerns in this disorder are associated globe rupture and increased pressure in the eye. Urgently evacuate these individuals. Place a protective shield over the eye. Restrict activity to walking only. Do not let these individuals read. Do not treat them with NSAIDs or aspirin because of the increased risk of bleeding.

Traumatic iritis may follow blunt trauma to the globe or a corneal abrasion. Keys to diagnosis are pain and photophobia following blunt trauma or after a corneal abrasion has healed. Traumatic iritis typically resolves without treatment in several days, but severe cases may be treated with topical prednisolone 1 percent drops four times a day for three days. Although topical steroids should not generally be prescribed except by ophthalmologists, use of prednisolone drops will probably not cause any significant adverse effects if given to an individual with a *fluorescein negative* eye disorder for no more than three days.

Not all ruptured globes are obvious. An occult ruptured globe may be suspected on the basis of severe blunt trauma, a history of an impaling injury or one that results from hammer fragmentation injury, the presence of dark uveal tissue exposed at the limbus, a distorted pupil, or a decrease in vision. An occult ruptured globe also entails the possibility of endophthalmitis and is treated in the same manner as an obvious open globe.

If there is no history of trauma, the next important diagnostic step is a fluorescein stain. Should this test reveal an epithelial defect, the diagnostic possibilities include a corneal ulcer, a corneal erosion, or herpes simplex keratitis. The mechanism for corneal ulcer occurrence in the absence of a history of trauma is usually contact lens wear. If a corneal ulcer is diagnosed based on an epithelial defect and a white or gray spot on the cornea, treat as described previously for a posttraumatic corneal ulcer. Discontinue contact lens wear in *both* eyes immediately and use glasses for refractive correction because the infection may be the result of contaminated lens solutions or cases.

The diagnosis of corneal erosion is made when there is an epithelial defect resembling a traumatic abrasion in the absence of a history of trauma. There is often a history of previous episodes. The onset of pain usually occurs when the eye is first opened in the morning. Treatment is as for a corneal abrasion. Corneal erosions are often slower to resolve than corneal abrasions because the sloughing epithelial tissue impedes healing of the corneal epithelium. The loose and mobile layer of sloughing corneal epithelium may need to be removed by a moistened cotton-tipped applicator after topical anesthesia if corneal healing is not progressing.

Herpes simplex keratitis is diagnosed by a typical dendritic figure on fluorescein staining and the absence of a history of trauma. There is often a history of previous episodes. Urgently evacuate a patient with this finding, since this disorder does not respond to topical antibiotics.

If the fluorescein stain reveals no epithelial defect, the next useful bit of diagnostic information is the response of the eye pain to topical anesthesia. Relief of eye pain by topical anesthesia indicates that the pain is due to an ocular surface disease (a discussion of some of these follows). If the pain is *not* relieved by topical anesthesia, then the next item of information needed is the size of the pupil in the affected eye compared to the fellow eye. If the pupil is dilated, then the likely diagnosis is angle-closure glaucoma (ACG). ACG usually occurs in patients older than forty and is accompanied by a decrease in vision and often by a history of previous episodes of eye pain. Treatment is with pilocarpine 2 percent, one drop every fifteen minutes for four doses in the affected eye, then four times a day in *both* eyes. Give acetazolamide 250 mg four times a day if available. Urgently evacuate the affected individual for definitive treatment with a laser iridotomy, since markedly elevated intraocular pressures may result in permanent damage to the optic nerve in twenty-four hours or less.

If the pain is *not* relieved by topical anesthesia, and the pupil is normal or constricted (miotic), then the likely diagnosis is either iritis or scleritis. Both diseases are often associated with systemic inflammatory disorders and may be vision threatening if not treated promptly and aggressively. Initiate treatment with prednisolone 1 percent, one drop every hour around the clock until evacuated. Also instill scopolamine 0.25 percent, one drop twice a day. The patient requires urgent evacuation. If improvement is not seen within twenty-four to forty-eight hours and evacuation has not been possible, start prednisone 80 mg once a day and continue until evacuation to definitive care is accomplished.

If the patient has no history of trauma, no epithelial defect, or no dendrites on fluorescein staining, and there is either no eye pain or the pain is significantly relieved by topical anesthesia, then the likely diagnosis is one of the following disorders.

1. Conjunctivitis

Conjunctivitis is recognized by an acute onset, the presence of an ocular discharge, exposure to other persons with eye infections, and/or upper respiratory infection symptoms. Treat with gatifloxacin 0.3 percent drops or moxifloxacin 0.5 percent drops, one drop four times a day for five days. Caution the affected individual about possible spread of the infection to the other eye as well as to other individuals. Note that many cases of conjunctivitis are of viral etiology and do not respond to antibiotics. Topical antibiotics should usually not be given for more than five days.

2. Blepharitis

This condition is often chronic, with a history of previous exacerbations and remissions. It is more common in older individuals and is usually bilateral, although one eye may be more severely affected than the other. Treatment is with bacitracin ointment applied to the lid margins once a day at bedtime for three to four weeks. One week of four-times-a-day application may be helpful in more severe cases. In addition, warm compresses used for ten minutes two to four times a day followed by gentle wiping away of the inflammatory material on the eyelashes is beneficial.

3. Ultraviolet keratitis

The diagnosis of UV keratitis, also known as snow blindness, is usually easy to make in the presence of bilateral eye pain and a sunburned face. As with sunburn of the skin, the symptoms do not reach their maximum intensity until several hours or longer after the exposure, so it is common for these patients to present in the evening hours. Fluorescein staining typically reveals no frank epithelial defect, but instead shows numerous small dots of stain uptake called superficial punctate keratitis (SPK). Treatment is with gatifloxacin/moxifloxacin drops four times a day until signs and symptoms resolve. These individuals are usually very photophobic, and sunglasses are helpful. Patch severely affected eyes for comfort, although it is usually better to avoid patching both eyes if possible, for obvious reasons. Scopolamine 0.25 percent, one drop twice a day, may be helpful in relieving pain if the discomfort merits the blurred vision and dilated pupil that scopolamine therapy entails. Systemic analgesia may be required. Monitor these individuals daily until epithelial staining resolves to ensure that they do not develop a corneal ulcer.

4. Foreign material in eye

Although the abrupt onset of a foreign-body sensation is strongly suggestive, definitive diagnosis requires identification of the foreign material, which
may sometimes be quite difficult. Treatment consists of location and removal
of the foreign body using enhanced lighting and magnification. Topical
anesthesia will make the patient much more comfortable during the
search and removal efforts, although it may be helpful to have the patient
identify the general location of the foreign material before applying topical anesthesia. Use a handheld magnifying lens or pair of reading glasses
to aid in the examination. Eyelid eversion with a cotton-tipped applicator will help the examiner to identify foreign bodies located on the upper
tarsal plate. Once the foreign body has been located, remove it with a
cotton-tipped applicator after the eye has been anesthetized and the cotton-
tipped applicator moistened with tetracaine. The eye is then stained with
fluorescein to check for a corneal abrasion. If no foreign body is visual-
ized, but symptoms persist, vigorous irrigation with artificial tears or sweeps
of the conjunctival fornices with a moistened cotton-tipped applicator after
topical anesthesia may be successful in removing the foreign body.

5. Dry eye

Symptomatic dry eye is commonly encountered in the wilderness, especially in mountainous areas where the air is very dry and significant wind
is often present. Dry eye is usually bilateral and may result in secondary
tearing. There may be a history of previous episodes of symptomatic dry
eye. Treatment is with artificial tears used as often as needed to relieve symptoms. Dehydration may contribute to this condition. The use of sunglasses may provide protection from the wind and be of significant benefit
in managing this disorder.

6. Contact lens overwear syndrome

Contact lens overwear syndrome may be another source of ocular discomfort in the wilderness. The considerations here are much as described
in the section on dry eye, except that the symptoms are magnified by the
presence of contact lenses. Contact lens rewetting drops and sunglasses
are the first line of management. Should these measures be ineffective in
relieving symptoms, remove the contact lenses. If significant SPK are
present on fluorescein staining, use gatifloxacin 0.3 percent drops or moxifloxacin 0.5 percent drops four times a day until the SPK have resolved.
Do not replace contact lenses until the eye is symptom-free. An individual who wears contact lenses in the wilderness should *always* carry a pair
of glasses that can be used if contact lens problems arise.

7. Episcleritis

Episcleritis is a generally benign and self-limited inflammation of the episclera (the lining of the eye between the conjunctiva and the sclera). There is usually sectoral redness without discharge and often a history of previous episodes. Discomfort is typically mild or absent. The presence of severe pain, photophobia, or decrease in vision suggests another diagnosis. Episcleritis is often misdiagnosed as conjunctivitis, but the lack of a discharge and the typical sectoral redness of episcleritis will help to differentiate between the two disorders. Episcleritis usually resolves without treatment over several weeks. If symptoms are troublesome, prednisolone 1 percent drops four times a day for three days may be used.

8. Subconjunctival hemorrhage

This condition may occur in the absence of trauma, often in association with coughing. Although the bright red appearance of the blood overlying the sclera may be alarming to the affected individual, this disorder is innocuous and will resolve without treatment over one to two weeks.

CHAPTER

10

High-Altitude Illness

Recommendations are considered Category 1B, except where indicated 1A, 2, or 3, by the WMS Panel of Expert Reviewers.

I. GENERAL INFORMATION

In unacclimatized persons ascending to high altitude, failure of the body to adapt to the stress of hypobaric hypoxia may lead to the cerebral and pulmonary syndromes of high-altitude illness. Acute mountain sickness (AMS) and high-altitude cerebral edema (HACE) refer to the cerebral disorders, and high-altitude pulmonary edema (HAPE) to the pulmonary abnormalities. High-altitude illnesses affect large numbers of wilderness travelers and result in occasional deaths. Proper management requires early diagnosis and prompt intervention. Most importantly, preventative measures such as gradual ascent will allow time for acclimatization and prevent high-altitude illness.

II. GUIDELINES FOR PREVENTION

Most altitude illness is preventable. The following measures reduce the incidence and severity of high-altitude illness. Although these measures do not guarantee freedom from illness, they are highly recommended, especially for those without altitude experience.

A. Staged ascent

The best strategy for prevention of acute mountain sickness is a gradual ascent to allow time for acclimatization (Category 1A). If possible, the first camp should be no higher than 8,000 feet (2,400 meters), with an increase of no more than 1,000 to 2,000 feet (300 to 600 meters) per night. An alternative approach is to spend two nights at the same altitude for every 2,000-

foot (600-meter) gain in altitude above 10,000 feet (3,000 meters). If a trip is started at over 9,000 feet (2,700 meters), two nights may be spent acclimatizing at that altitude before proceeding higher. Proceed higher during the day and return to a lower elevation to sleep (climb high, sleep low).

B. High-carbohydrate diet

A significant energy deficit may occur after ascent to high altitude because appetite is suppressed, food may be less available or less palatable, and energy expenditure is increased. Nutritional intake should be increased by about 500 kcal per day above appetite, emphasizing carbohydrate-rich foods, which may aid acclimatization and prevent altitude illness (Category 2).

C. Appropriate exercise level

Until acclimatized, exercise moderately, avoiding excessive dyspnea and fatigue.

D. Hydration

To offset increased fluid losses at high altitudes, stay well hydrated. Adequate hydration may be judged by the presence of clear urine. In the setting of established high-altitude illness, however, forced overhydration should be avoided because it may increase fluid retention and worsen symptoms (Category 2).

E. Drug prophylaxis

Several drugs can lessen the symptoms of high-altitude illness. In general, use of drugs to prevent high-altitude illness is reserved for those persons with a prior history on previous ascents.

1. Acetazolamide

Effective for prophylaxis of AMS (Category 1A). The indications for acetazolamide prophylaxis are a forced rapid ascent, proceeding to sleeping altitude greater than about 9,000 feet (2,700 meters) in one day from less than 3,500 feet (1,000 meters), or a history of previous AMS at similar rates of ascent. Acetazolamide is considered the drug of choice for chemoprophylaxis of AMS.

The dose of acetazolamide for adults is 250 mg twice a day, starting the day before ascent. The dose for children is 4 mg/kg a day.

Common side effects from this drug include peripheral paresthesias, altered taste, and polyuria. As this drug is a diuretic, the increase in urine fluid loss needs to be replaced. Contraindications are pregnancy, metabolic or respiratory acidosis, or allergy to sulfa drugs. Myopia is rare and reversible with cessation.

2. Dexamethasone

May be used to prevent AMS (Category 1A) either for those who cannot take acetazolamide, or for a forced rapid ascent to very high altitude, such as flying to over 14,000 feet (4,250 meters) on an overnight rescue.

The dosage for adults is 4 mg orally every six to eight hours. Starting the medication two to four hours prior to ascent is probably adequate, although the exact timing for beginning and discontinuing the medication has not yet been established. Discontinuing dexamethasone before acclimatization has taken place may "unmask" the symptoms of AMS.

Dyspepsia, bizarre dreams, dysphoria, and euphoria occasionally occur. On longer treks or expeditions it is more problematic to start and stop dexamethasone as compared to acetazolamide because of the potential effects on the adrenal axis.

3. Ginkgo biloba

A newer, and more controversial, alternative for pharmacological prophylaxis of AMS (Category 3). Studies have been conflicting regarding efficacy. In small, randomized, controlled studies ginkgo biloba has been found to be effective in preventing AMS and in reducing severity. In a larger study comparing ginkgo biloba to acetazolamide in prevention of AMS in a Himalayan trekking population, however, ginkgo biloba was not effective, but acetazolamide (250 mg twice daily) was effective. At this point, the efficacy of ginkgo biloba for prevention of AMS remains uncertain, and further studies are required. Doses used in the studies are 80 to 120 mg by mouth two times a day starting five days before ascent. Ginkgo biloba may increase bleeding risk in persons on anticoagulant or antiplatelet drugs, otherwise there are essentially no side effects.

4. Nifedipine

The prophylactic administration of nifedipine is effective in lowering pulmonary artery pressure and preventing high-altitude pulmonary edema in HAPE-susceptible individuals. The prophylactic dose of nifedipine is 30 or 60 mg (extended release formation) per day to be taken during the ascent phase of the expedition and for three additional days at altitude.

Possible side effects include those of orthostatic hypotension, although the drug is very well tolerated in persons with normal cardiovascular function. Consider the use of this drug as an adjunct to the most important preventive measure, gradual ascent.

5. Inhaled salmeterol

Effective in increasing fluid clearance from alveoli and preventing HAPE. The dose studied is 125 micrograms inhaled twice daily, which is two to three times the recommended dose for asthma. Potential side effects are those of systemic beta-agonist adrenergic stimulation and include anxiety, tachycardia, and tremor. There is less experience with the use of inhaled salmeterol as compared to nifedipine for prophylaxis of HAPE. Both drugs could be used simultaneously, but both are considered as adjuncts to gradual ascent.

F. Sedatives and hypnotics

Medications to aid sleep at high altitude include acetazolamide and benzodiazepines. Acetazolamide has the advantage of aiding acclimatization by causing a metabolic acidosis with compensatory hyperventilation, thus augmenting the normal increased ventilation and respiratory alkalosis that occurs during acclimatization. Acetazolamide also has the advantage of eliminating sleep period breathing (Cheyne-Stokes), which is universal above about 13,000 feet. Benzodiazepines are effective sleeping medications at high altitude in persons who are healthy, but they may be harmful in those who have high-altitude illness because suppressing respirations may lead to worse hypoxemia during sleep and acceleration of high-altitude illness.

III. GUIDELINES FOR ASSESSMENT AND TREATMENT

Ascending too quickly and not allowing time for acclimatization increases susceptibility to high-altitude illness. Descent is a treatment for all forms of high-altitude illness and may be lifesaving for HAPE or HACE (Category 1A). Mild forms of AMS, however, usually resolve spontaneously in two to four days if ascent is halted, making descent unnecessary. There are few studies of treatment of AMS, and these guidelines reflect expert opinion more than well-controlled research studies. Treatment is based on four principles:

■ Stop ascent in presence of symptoms (do not go up unless symptoms go away).
■ Descend if there is no improvement or condition worsens.
■ Descend immediately if symptoms of HAPE or HACE are present.
■ Ill persons must not be left alone or sent down alone.

A. Acute mountain sickness

Individuals with AMS have headache and at least one other symptom of anorexia, nausea, vomiting, dizziness, lightheadedness, disturbed sleep, or lassitude. There are no characteristic physical findings. Basic treatment is to descend or to stop ascent and wait for improvement before proceeding. Continuing ascent in the presence of symptoms is ill-advised. After stopping the ascent, more advanced treatment consists of administering supplemental oxygen by nasal cannula at a flow to achieve an arterial oxygen saturation (SaO_2 percent) of greater than 90 percent as measured by a digital pulse oximeter, or about 2 liters per minute flow if measurement of oxygen saturation is not available. Oxygen may be especially helpful during sleep. Aspirin or acetaminophen, with hydrocodone if necessary, are useful for headache. Prochlorperazine or promethazine can be used for nausea. Prochlorperazine 10 mg parenterally or orally every six hours, or 25 mg rectally every twelve hours, for an average-size adult, also increases the hypoxic drive to breathe. Promethazine can be administered as 25 mg parenterally, or as 25 or 50 mg suppositories for adults every eight hours. Use no more than three doses of either drug. Note that both prochlorperazine and promethazine may cause extrapyramidal reactions requiring treatment with diphenhydramine. Treatment of the illness, rather than just the symptoms, requires acetazolamide. The treatment dose is 250 mg twice a day. Acetazolamide speeds acclimatization and aborts the illness. An alternative for persons who are sulfa allergic is dexamethasone 4 mg every six to eight hours. A response is usually seen within twelve to twenty-four hours. If the illness progresses, descent is mandatory.

B. High-altitude pulmonary edema

Mild HAPE presents with decreased exercise performance, fatigue, dyspnea on exertion while moving uphill, a dry cough, and localized inspiratory crackles on lung auscultation. In moderate to severe HAPE there is marked weakness and fatigue, dyspnea on exertion walking on level ground, a cough of scant sputum that progresses to frothy pink sputum, tachypnea, tachycardia, a gurgling sensation in the chest, and bilateral inspiratory crackles on lung auscultation. Hypoxemia is present as measured by an SaO_2 percent lower than normal for a given altitude. Neurological symptoms and signs may also be present.

In a wilderness or mountaineering situation, descent is the primary treatment. Descending 2,000 to 4,000 feet (600 to 1,200 meters) often results in marked improvement in symptoms, but descent should continue until medical care is reached or symptoms resolve. Persons with HAPE should be accompanied by a healthy member of the party and should not be left alone. Oxygen, if available, is a useful adjunct to descent and improves arterial oxygenation, lowers pulmonary arterial pressure, and improves symptoms. Oxygen may be used as the primary treatment without descent in settings where supplemental oxygen is available around the clock and medical care is nearby—such as at ski resorts. Flow of oxygen should be sufficient to raise SaO_2 to 90 percent or greater.

Adjuncts to oxygen and descent include nifedipine 10 mg orally or sublingual every four hours or 30 or 60 mg sustained release once a day. An expiratory positive airway pressure (EPAP) mask can be a temporizing measure. A portable hyperbaric bag may be lifesaving when descent is impossible by providing a physiologic descent of about 5,000 feet when pressurized. Constant monitoring of a patient in a portable hyperbaric bag is mandatory. Treatment continues until symptoms resolve or the weather or climbing conditions permit the aided descent of the patient. One strategy for treatment of HAPE in a portable hyperbaric bag is fifty minutes inside the bag followed by a ten-minute break every hour.

C. High-altitude cerebral edema

HACE is characterized by progressive neurological deterioration with a headache and change in the level of consciousness associated with ataxia, progressing to obtundation and eventually coma. Immediate descent is mandatory until obvious improvement occurs. Oxygen and dexamethasone are recommended as adjunctive therapy with descent. Supplemental oxygen is titrated to achieve an SaO_2 of 90 percent or greater. Be observant for concomitant HAPE. Dexamethasone 8–12 mg is given immediately by the route most easily available, followed by 4 mg every six hours until symptoms subside. Response is usually noted within twelve to twenty-four hours, but descent is still mandatory, and ataxia may be slow to resolve even after descent and treatment with oxygen and dexamethasone. Hospitalization is commonly required after evacuation from high altitude, and treatment may include endotracheal intubation for airway protection and treatment of increased intracranial pressure. If descent is not possible in a field setting because of weather or terrain conditions, then a portable hyperbaric bag may be used to simulate descent as a temporizing measure.

D. Peripheral edema

High altitudes may cause swelling of the hands, ankles, or face (usually the periorbital region). Elevate the extremities, if possible. The edema will resolve with descent, but descent is not mandatory unless signs and symptoms of more serious altitude illnesses are present.

E. High-altitude retinopathy

Retinal hemorrhages are common above 16,000 feet (5,000 meters) but may develop at lower altitudes. They are generally asymptomatic and do not warrant descent or other treatment. However, when a retinal hemorrhage overlies the macula, it may cause blindness. They usually resolve after descent, although a blind spot may persist for years or permanently.

REFERENCES

Reviews supporting all Category 1A recommendations

Bartsch, P., and R. Roach. 2001. Acute mountain sickness and high-altitude cerebral edema. In High altitude, an exploration of human adaptation, ed. T. F. Hornbein and R. B. Schoene, from *Lung biology in health and disease,* ed. C. Lenfant, 731–76. New York: Marcel Dekker, Inc.

Grissom, C. K., and R. B. Schoene. 2004. Adaptation and maladaptation to high altitude. In *Baum's textbook of pulmonary diseases,* 7th ed., ed. J. D. Crapo, J. Glassroth, J. Karlinsky, and T. E. King, 1,005–23. Philadelphia: Lippincott Williams & Wilkins.

Hackett, P. H., and R. C. Roach. 2001. High altitude illness. *N Engl J Med* 345:107–14.

———. 2001. High altitude medicine. In *Wilderness Medicine*, 4th ed., P. S. Auerbach, 2–43. St. Louis, Mo.: Mosby.

Schoene, R. B., P. H. Hackett, and T. F. Hornbein. 2000. High altitude. In *Textbook of respiratory medicine,* 3rd ed., ed. J. F. Murray and J. A. Nadel, 1,915–950. New York: W. B. Saunders Co.

Studies supporting Category 1A recommendation of gradual ascent for prevention of high-altitude illness

Hackett, P. H., D. Rennie, and H. D. Levine. 1976. The incidence, importance, and prophylaxis of acute mountain sickness. *Lancet* 2:1,149–155.

Hackett, P. H., and I. D. Rennie. 1979. Rales, peripheral edema, retinal hemorrhage and acute mountain sickness. *Am J Med* 67:214–18.

Purkayastha, S. S., U. S. Ray, B. S. Arora, et al. 1995. Acclimatization at high altitude in gradual and acute induction. *J Appl Physiol* 79:487–92.

Singh, I., P. K. Khanna, M. C. Srivastava, et al. 1969. Acute mountain sickness. *New Engl J Med* 280:175–84.

Studies supporting Category 1A recommendation of acetazolamide for AMS prophylaxis

Basnyat, B., J. H. Gertsch, E. W. Johnson, et al. 2003. Efficacy of low-dose acetazolamide (125 mg BID) for the prophylaxis of acute mountain sickness: A prospective, double-blind, randomized placebo-controlled trial. *High Alt Med Biol* 4:45–52.

Dumont, L., C. Mardirosoff, and M. R. Tramer. 2000. Efficacy and harm of pharmacological prevention of acute mountain sickness: Quantitative systematic review. *BMJ* 321:267–72.

Gertsch, J. H., B. Basnyat, E. W. Johnson, et al. 2004. Randomized, double blind, placebo controlled comparison of ginkgo biloba and acetazolamide for prevention of acute mountain sickness among Himalayan trekkers: The prevention of high altitude illness trial (PHAIT). *BMJ* 7443:797.

Gray, G. W., A. C. Bryan, R. Frayser, et al. 1971. Control of acute mountain sickness. *Aerosp Med* 42:81–84.

Greene, M. K., A. M. Kerr, I. B. McIntosh, and R. J. Prescott. 1981. Acetazolamide in prevention of acute mountain sickness: A double blind controlled cross-over study. *Br Med J* (Clin Res Ed) 283:811–13.

Larson, E. B., R. C. Roach, R. B. Schoene, and T. F. Hornbein. 1982. Acute mountain sickness and acetazolamide: Clinical efficacy and effect on ventilation. *JAMA* 248:328–32.

Studies supporting Category 1A recommendation of dexamethasone for AMS prophylaxis

Bernhard, W. N., L. M. Schalick, P. A. Delaney, et al. 1998. Acetazolamide plus low-dose dexamethasone is better than acetazolamide alone to ameliorate symptoms of acute mountain sickness. *Aviat Space Environ Med* 69:883–86.

Ellsworth, A. J., E. F. Meyer, and E. B. Larson. 1991. Acetazolamide or dexamethasone use versus placebo to prevent acute mountain sickness on Mt. Rainier. *West J Med* 154:289–93.

Ellsworth, A. J., E. B. Larson, and D. Strickland. 1987. A randomized trial of dexamethasone and acetazolamide for acute mountain sickness prophylaxis. *Am J Med* 83:1,024.

Hackett, P. H., R. C. Roach, R. A. Wood, et al. 1988. Dexamethasone for prevention and treatment of acute mountain sickness. *Aviat Space Environ Med* 59:950–54.

Johnson, T. S., P. B. Rock, C. S. Fulco, et al. 1984. Prevention of acute mountain sickness by dexamethasone. *N Engl J Med* 310:683–86.

Rock, P. B., T. S. Johnson, R. F. Larsen, et al. 1989. Dexamethasone as prophylaxis for acute mountain sickness, effect of dose level. *Chest* 95:568–73.

Zell, S. C., and P. H. Goodman. 1988. Acetazolamide and dexamethasone in the prevention of acute mountain sickness. *West J Med* 148:541–45.

Hypothermia

Recommendations are considered Category 1B, except where indicated 1A, by the WMS Panel of Expert Reviewers.

I. GENERAL INFORMATION

Hypothermia occurs when the body's ability to generate and conserve heat is overcome by heat loss. **Acute** hypothermia presents with a sudden drop in body core temperature within a few hours. This is usually caused by immersion in cold water or a sudden drop in ambient temperature combined with wind and precipitation. **Chronic** hypothermia is the result of a gradual drop in body core temperature over several hours. Most chronic hypothermia deaths occur when the ambient temperature ranges from 30 to 50°F (-1 to 10°C). Hypothermia is almost always preventable by minimizing heat loss via conduction, convection, radiation, and evaporation. Prevention includes:

- Proper choice and use of clothing and shelter
- Avoidance of overexertion
- Staying dry (a combination of proper clothing and avoidance of overexertion)
- Staying well hydrated
- Maintenance of adequate nutrition

A. Mild hypothermia

Hypothermia is considered mild if the core temperature is below 95°F (35°C) and above 90°F (32°C). In this temperature range, the thermoregulatory defense mechanisms, such as shivering, are generally unimpaired and operating maximally. Mild hypothermia often first manifests itself as loss of judgment and fine motor coordination. Shivering is often suppressed by physical activity, but by the time core temperature reaches 95°F (35°C), most patients are shivering vigorously. Uncontrollable shivering will be seen during further cooling to 90°F (32°C), except in some chronic exposure situations (longer than six to eight hours) where exhaustion and shivering fatigue may occur. Slurred speech, a stumbling gait, and the development of ataxia are highly suggestive of hypothermia in a cold-exposed patient. It is important to note that most patients with mild hypothermia are fully able to rewarm themselves through shivering heat production, although they require protection from further heat loss in order to do so. The exception will be an exhausted patient who is unable to shiver.

B. Moderate to severe hypothermia

Hypothermia is considered moderate at core temperatures below 90°F (32°C) and above 82°F (28°C), and severe at core temperatures below 82°F (28°C).

Since taking core temperature measurements may not be possible or appropriate in the field, diagnosis can be based on observations and functional characteristics.

As core temperature decreases within the moderate range, thermoregulatory shivering is progressively inhibited until it stops and the patient loses the ability to rewarm (usually at a core temperature of about 86°F (30°C). The patient may have a profoundly altered mental status, loss of coordination, lassitude, and an apathetic attitude. Finally, consciousness will be lost.

As core temperature decreases below 82°F (28°C) (severe hypothermia), the heart is at risk of ventricular fibrillation either spontaneously due to low heart temperature or as a reflex response to mechanical stimulation. The patient loses consciousness, and pupils may be dilated and fixed. The torso will be cold to the touch. The patient may be rigid and unresponsive, with nonpalpable pulse and respirations, but not dead (the patient cannot be presumed dead unless these conditions persist after warming, or if obvious signs of fatal trauma are present).

II. GUIDELINES FOR FIELD TREATMENT
A. General principles

The general principles of treatment apply for all cases of hypothermia. The patient must be gently removed from the cold exposure and remain in a horizontal position. *Remove wet clothing carefully and insulate the patient completely* (e.g., with one or even two sleeping bags) while maintaining an adequate exposure of the airways. This will minimize convective and conductive heat loss. A vapor barrier (e.g., plastic sheet, space blanket, etc.) can be added to eliminate evaporative heat loss and *protect the insulation from becoming wet*. If wet clothing cannot be removed safely, place the vapor barrier between the clothing and insulation. If the patient is dry, the barrier could be placed outside the insulation.

B. Mild hypothermia

A mildly hypothermic patient will normally be shivering vigorously and may be dehydrated. Administer fuel for shivering with warm high-energy drinks (nonalcoholic) and foods, providing the patient is alert and can swallow without choking.

External heat sources, such as chemical or charcoal heat packs and hot-water bottles, can be used. For rewarming purposes, the heat should be applied preferentially to the chest and armpits. During winter transport heat should be applied to the soles of the feet to prevent frostbite (*provided frostbite is not already present*). Place the palms of the hands on the chest. Do not apply these heat sources directly to the patient's skin, but over a thin layer of clothing.

Exercise will generate heat but may also precipitate a significant drop in core temperature (afterdrop). If the patient is otherwise healthy and vigorously shivering, mild exercise may be initiated only after forty-five to sixty minutes of shivering in an insulated environment. At this point the afterdrop should be reversed. However, if any deterioration in physical or mental condition occurs during exercise, it should stop immediately.

C. Moderate to severe hypothermia

Whether a patient is moderately or severely hypothermic, the clinical condition is serious: Treatment is the same *under all circumstances.* The patient must be handled very gently and kept in the horizontal position. Because of the risk of inducing ventricular fibrillation, remove wet clothing and take care to minimize patient movement while performing other life-sustaining measures. Make arrangements to transfer the patient to medical facilities as soon as possible.

Shivering will be weak, intermittent, or nonexistent, and the patient will not rewarm spontaneously. The condition may degenerate progressively. Application of moderate heat to the chest and armpits is indicated. Place external heat sources, such as heat packs, etc., over a thin layer of clothing as previously indicated.

Warmed and humidified supplemental oxygen may be administered. This is unlikely to significantly heat the body core; however, improvement in cardiovascular and mental function has been reported with this treatment, likely due to rewarming of the brainstem via heat transfer form the upper airways.

Do not give a patient with impaired consciousness any warm drinks as this may cause burns and/or choking. Aggressive rewarming, such as warm-water immersion, should never be attempted as this may cause ventricular fibrillation. Do not rub the extremities under any condition—rubbing produces little frictional heat and damages the skin and underlying tissue (especially if it is frozen).

D. Cardiopulmonary resuscitation

A cold, rigid, apparently pulseless and breathless patient is not necessarily a dead patient. A cold patient with no detectable pulse should not necessarily be given chest compressions. Apparent pulselessness may be caused by hypothermia and the resulting tissue rigidity in combination with a very slow heart rate. Under these conditions chest compressions may trigger ventricular fibrillation and will not be effective in someone dead from the cold.

Check for breathing and pulse for a full minute, because vital signs in hypothermia may be present but very slow and faint. If you fail to detect cardiac activity or respiration, initiate rescue breathing immediately. This should continue for three minutes as improved oxygenation may strengthen cardiac activity and make it detectable. The patient needs oxygen, and there is *no* danger to the patient from rescue breathing. If bag and mask are used (with ambient air or compressed oxygen), care should be taken not to hyperventilate the patient as the heart is more susceptible to fibrillation during periods of hypocarbia. After three minutes of rescue breathing, another sixty seconds should be taken to detect cardiac activity and respiration. If the patient is still pulseless and breathless, chest compressions could be initiated.

Do not initiate chest compressions in a patient who has been submerged in cold water for more than one hour, has a core temperature of less than 10°C, has obvious fatal injuries, is frozen (e.g., ice formation in the airway), has a chest wall that is so stiff that compressions are impossible, or if the rescuers are exhausted or in danger (Category 1A) (reference: State of Alaska Cold Injuries Guidelines, revised 11/2003).

Defibrillation is rarely effective if the core temperature is below 30°C (Category 1A) (reference: Danzl, D. F. 2001. Accidental hypothermia. In *Wilderness medicine,* 4th ed., ed. P. S. Auerbach, 152. St. Louis, Mo.: Mosby, Inc.).

In the patient who is not breathing and has no pulse, the clinical decisions are based on access to transportation:

■ If transportation is available within three hours, begin ventilation (intubate if possible), protect from further cooling, and do not start chest compressions. Wait for the rescue crew. Starting chest compressions might precipitate ventricular fibrillation in a patient who actually has a weak pulse, which is difficult to detect, but which might be providing adequate perfusion. If chest compressions cause ventricular fibrillation, perfusion will be lost.

■ If transportation is not available within three hours, begin ventilation (intubate if possible), start chest compressions, and perform for up to thirty minutes while attempting to rewarm the patient. If this is unsuccessful in restoring spontaneous circulation, discontinue CPR.

■ Performing CPR while litter bearing is not effective and should not be attempted (Category 1A) (reference: State of Alaska Cold Injuries Guidelines, revised 11/2003).

III. GUIDELINES FOR EVACUATION

If a patient with mild hypothermia is adequately rewarmed, with a return to normal mental status, there is no need for evacuation. Take care to prevent a recurrence. Monitor the patient while walking with him/her to the nearest location where treatment is practical. Patients who do not respond to rewarming, or who obviously have moderate to severe hypothermia, must be insulated for maximum heat retention, provided with moderate heat source(s), and be evacuated as soon as possible. Evacuation of such a patient must be as gentle as possible to prevent ventricular fibrillation. Package the person so that rescue personnel are able to examine the patient periodically. Every fifteen minutes during transport check the patient for:

■ Vital signs
■ Burning of the skin underneath heat sources
■ Circulation in the feet to examine for frostbite, unless this examination increases heat loss, in which case be judicious in monitoring as often as practical

12

Frostbite/Immersion Foot

Recommendations are considered Category 1B by the WMS Panel of Expert Reviewers.

I. GENERAL INFORMATION

Frostbite is localized injury or death of tissue from exposure to subfreezing cold. The chance of damage is increased by:

- Temperatures 24°F (-4.5°C) or below
- High winds
- High altitude
- Use of tobacco, alcohol, or other drugs
- Contact with heat-conductive materials, such as metal, water, or gasoline
- Overexertion, which produces fatigue and sweat
- Previous frostbite injury
    Measures to help prevent frostbite include:
- Avoiding tight boots or too many pairs of socks in larger boots
- Preserving heat by keeping head, neck, and face covered
- Wearing mittens instead of gloves
- Staying well hydrated
- Maintaining metabolic heat production with adequate caloric intake
- Keeping dry
- Avoiding direct skin-metal or skin-fluid contact

    Immersion foot (trenchfoot) is a cold weather, nonfreezing injury resulting from vasoconstriction of the arterioles with subsequent loss of heat and oxygen supply to surface tissues. Prevention includes:

- Avoidance of tightly fitting footwear
- Changing into dry socks regularly (at least once a day)

■ Periodic (every four hours in extreme wet and cold conditions) air-drying, elevation, and massaging of feet to promote circulation

---

II. GUIDELINES FOR ASSESSMENT AND TREATMENT

A. Superficial frostbite (frostnip)

A small patch of skin is white, but it rapidly returns to normal with warm breath or skin-to-skin rewarming. No special treatment required.

B. Partial thickness frostbite

The skin is pale, cold, and numb, but underlying tissues remain soft and pliable. Treat superficial frostbite with passive skin-to-skin contact or rapid rewarming, but avoid heat exposure greater than 108°F (42°C). After thawing, a few clear fluid-filled blisters develop in superficial frostbite. If damage is extensive, blisters may fill with bloody fluid, and treatment should be administered as in deep frostbite (see C). Extreme care must be taken with frostbitten tissue to prevent refreezing. Evacuate as soon as possible if blisters have formed. This can be a self-evacuation if the hands are involved, but it might require a litter evacuation if the feet are affected. Give ibuprofen every six hours to inhibit thromboxane production. Maintain adequate hydration. Protect blisters with clean gauze or a cloth bandage.

C. Full thickness (deep) frostbite

Skin and deep structures, including muscle, tendons, and possibly even bone, are involved. The affected part is hard and not pliable. On diagnosis of deep frostbite, evacuate patient immediately. Patients with frostbitten, unthawed feet may walk to self-evacuate. During evacuation, if possible, protect the affected part with dry insulation, such as clean dry socks or dry mittens. Remove jewelry and all constrictive clothing. After evacuation, or if transportation is certain, rapidly rewarm the frostbitten area in water preheated to 100.4 to 104°F (38 to 40°C). After thawing, multiple fluid-filled and hemorrhagic blisters form. The portion of the extremity beyond the hemorrhagic blisters is extremely damaged and may eventually become mummified over time. Suspend the frostbitten area in the container of water without allowing contact with the sides. Check water temperature often. Avoid excessive heat. During thawing, pain is usually severe, and analgesics, including narcotics, are indicated. When rewarming is accomplished, dry the affected parts gently, and place sterile gauze between digits. Elevate the injured part. Give ibuprofen every six hours to inhibit thromboxane production. Maintain adequate hydration. Provide definitive medical care as soon as possible.

D. Immersion foot

Injury includes cold, swollen, waxy feet, mottled with dark burgundy to blue splotches. Skin is sodden and friable. In the later stage, feet become red and hot, and blisters often form. Infection and gangrene frequently result. Field treatment includes:

- Maintenance of dry, warm feet
- Oral hydration
- Ibuprofen every six hours to inhibit thromboxane production
- Immediate evacuation to definitive care (*NOTE:* walking may be difficult for the patient)

III. CONTROVERSIES

Should deep frostbite be thawed in the field?

There is evidence that the longer tissue stays frozen, the worse the injury. Frozen extremities in an otherwise uninjured patient are difficult to keep frozen, and spontaneous thawing usually occurs during evacuation. Field therapy, which can render an ambulatory patient nonambulatory, must be balanced against the time required for evacuation.

Should a patient self-evacuate on frozen toes/feet prior to thawing if worse freezing is unlikely or field thawing cannot be easily accomplished?

The longer the extremity is frozen, the greater the tissue damage, although even more significant damage occurs with a thaw followed by freezing. The decision to walk out on frozen feet should not be made if there is any reasonable ability to thaw and provide further protection from freezing. Thawed toes may not be so painful as to preclude self-evacuation. Deep frostbite of the entire foot may become so painful and debilitating upon thawing that self-evacuation becomes impossible. As the field diagnosis before thawing may be difficult to accurately assess, frozen extremities should generally be thawed and protected from further freezing as soon as possible, with the knowledge that the victim might not be able to self-evacuate.

CHAPTER

13

Heat-Related Illnesses

Recommendations are considered Category 1B by the WMS Panel of Expert Reviewers.

I. GENERAL INFORMATION

Heat-related illnesses comprise several conditions caused by exposure to hot environments, or intense exercise in moderate environments, that range from mild discomfort to life-threatening illness. Hyperthermia occurs when heat stress on the body, from internal metabolic heat production and external sources, overcomes the heat dissipating capability of the body. Extreme or untreated hyperthermia can rapidly become life-threatening.

Heat illnesses are preventable. Prevention includes:

- **Acclimatization.** The process by which the body adapts to heat exposure, acclimatization is induced by a minimum of sixty to ninety minutes of exercise in the heat each day for one to two weeks. Initial adaptation occurs within a few days. The most significant change is an increase in sweat volume initiated at a lower skin temperature. This increases evaporative cooling and results in a lower heart rate and core temperature for a given amount of work in the heat.
- **Hydration with adequate fluid quantities.** An acclimatized person can lose 1 L/h or greater of sweat during exercise. Relieving thirst alone risks not maintaining full hydration. Start each work period by drinking 500 ml of water. At least 300–500 ml per hour is then likely to be required, and requirements may be higher with extreme exertion or sweat loss (see chapter 16). In extreme conditions, sweat loss may exceed gastric emptying, and intravenous fluids may be required.
- **Appropriate clothing.** Dress appropriately in light-colored, loose-fitting clothing, allowing maximum evaporative heat loss.
- **Frequent rest.** Rest frequently, especially before full acclimatization, preferably in shade during the hottest part of the day.

- **Maximization of evaporative cooling.** Periodically dip clothing in water, if possible.
- **Physical fitness.** This improves the rate and quality of acclimatization, but it does not provide heat adaptation by itself. The insulation of excess body fat reduces heat loss.

II. GUIDELINES FOR ASSESSMENT AND TREATMENT

A. Heat cramps

Heat cramps are muscle spasms that may be severe, usually in large, heavily exercised muscle groups like legs and abdomen. They are probably caused by a combination of electrolyte depletion, hyperventilation with respiratory alkalosis, and plasma volume depletion. Rest the patient and give oral or intravenous fluids that contain sodium. Cold oral fluids are absorbed more quickly than warm ones. Gentle stretching of the cramped muscles is usually beneficial. After recovery, the activity may be resumed, but if the cramps return, a twenty-four-hour rest is recommended.

B. Heat syncope

Heat syncope is seen immediately after periods of strenuous work in hot environments. Patients regain consciousness quickly. Treat with recumbent rest in a cooler area and splash water with fanning to enhance cooling. Oral rehydration is indicated when fully alert. Assess the patient for injuries if a fall was associated with the syncope.

C. Heat rash

Heat rash (prickly heat, or miliaria) is an acute inflammatory disease of the skin seen in humid regions following prolonged sweating. Sweat-gland ducts become blocked with keratinizing cells, and accumulated sweat is forced through the duct walls, inciting inflammation in adjacent soft tissue. Erythematous pruritic papules appear on trunk and extremities, excluding hands and feet. Secondary infection may occur. In severe cases, heat tolerance is reduced due to decreased sweating. In the field, keep the affected areas clean and limit exercise and heat exposure.

D. Heat exhaustion

Heat exhaustion is caused by dehydration and intravascular volume depletion in a thermally stressful environment. Symptoms and signs include: weakness, inability to work, headache, mild confusion, nausea, faintness, anorexia, dyspnea, and rapid pulse. Skin may be warm or cool with sweating. The core temperature may be normal or moderately elevated. In practice, the distinction between heat exhaustion and heat stroke may be somewhat blurred. Should doubt exist, then always err on the side of caution and treat as per heat stroke (see E). Otherwise, remove the patient to a cooler area, allow to rest, and rehydrate orally, preferably with cold, lightly salted water or an electrolyte solution. The patient may benefit from cooling of the skin by wetting and fanning. When the patient has fully recovered, the activity may continue. Depending on the extent of the illness, recovery may take as long as twenty-four hours.

E. Heat stroke

Heat stroke (both classical from exposure to heat and exertional from work in heat) are true medical emergencies in which elevated core body temperature (above 105°F [40.5°C] rectally) causes renal, hepatic, and nervous system damage. Persons at an increased risk of heat stroke include those who are obese, unfit, unacclimatized, elderly, acutely ill, or dehydrated from vomiting or diarrhea; individuals with underlying medical conditions, such as coronary heart disease and hyperthyroidism; and individuals on certain medications, such as beta-blockers, stimulants, diuretics, or anticholinergics.

Skin may be dry or sweating preserved, especially in a fit person suffering exertional heat stroke. Symptoms and signs include confusion, disorientation, bizarre behavior, ataxia, tachycardia, tachypnea, and hot, red skin. Both heat stroke and heat exhaustion may present as collapse in the face of a heat load—environmental heat, metabolic heat from exercise, or a combination of both. Both may have altered consciousness, elevated temperatures, and rapid pulse. Heat stroke is differentiated from heat exhaustion by the presence of cardiovascular shock, persistent profound mental status changes, and markedly elevated temperature. In heat exhaustion, mental status and blood pressure normalize rapidly as in syncope, if the patient is recumbent in the shade.

Heat stroke has a high mortality rate. Whenever there is altered mental status and elevated temperature, rapid cooling is essential and must be started in the field. Treatment may include:
- Shading from direct sunlight and removal of clothing
- Wetting with tepid or cool water and fanning aggressively
- Placing ice packs at the neck, armpits, and groin
- Performing cold water immersion (the most efficient cooling method), if possible
- Giving intravenous fluids, if possible

If possible, check the rectal temperature every five to ten minutes and, when the temperature reaches approximately 100 to 102°F (37.7 to 38.8°C), taper off the cooling efforts, as rapid cooling below this point may lead to shivering. If the patient returns to a level of consciousness appropriate for oral hydration, give fluids. Do not give antipyretics such as aspirin or acetaminophen. Rapid evacuation is indicated. Monitor carefully for rebound temperature increase.

CHAPTER

14

Lightning Injuries

Recommendations are considered Category 1B by the WMS Panel of Expert Reviewers.

I. GENERAL INFORMATION

One bolt of lightning may generate 300,000 amps and 2 billion volts—an awesome power capable of great destructive force. A single strike often injures or kills more than one person. Lightning injures or kills in one of the following ways:

■ Direct strike
■ Splash after striking a nearby object
■ Ground current
■ Trauma from the blast of exploding air
■ Direct contact with an object carrying current

Lightning causes serious injury or death in about one-third of its victims and permanent sequelae of some sort in about two-thirds of survivors. The factors related to a fatal outcome include immediate cardiopulmonary arrest, acute neurologic and/or traumatic injuries, or leg or head burns. Because any electrical current takes the shortest path between contact points, multiple organ systems may be injured. The duration of a lightning strike is so brief (less than one millisecond) that it may not penetrate, but "flash over" the patient's skin.

Although lightning strikes are unpredictable, there are ways to reduce the chance of injury. During an electrical storm:

■ Avoid open areas where you are one of the tallest objects.
■ Do not seek shelter under a single tree, bush, or rock that stands in an open area.
■ Avoid extremes of high or low ground.
■ Avoid contact with metal objects.
■ Seek shelter deep in a dry cave, staying away from the sides and roof.

- Seek shelter among trees or bushes or rocks of uniform size.
- If boating, attempt to get to shore, waves and shoreline permitting.
- Squat with your feet close together or sit in a compact position on a nonconductive material, such as a foam pad or rope coil.
- Spread out a group but stay close enough to maintain visual contact with each other.

II. GUIDELINES FOR ASSESSMENT

Victims of lightning strikes are not electrically charged and pose no threat to rescuers. Patients typically fall into one of three categories:

- Minimally injured, requiring little immediate care other than psychological support, although they must receive a thorough examination when time allows
- Seriously injured, often initially unconscious, requiring immediate attention to airway and obvious injuries, including appropriate stabilization for possible head and spine injuries
- Maximally injured, in cardiopulmonary arrest

Initiate rescue breathing and chest compressions (CPR) immediately on all pulseless, breathless victims of lightning strike. Following a severe electrical shock, respiratory paralysis may persist long after cardiac activity returns. Rescuers must be prepared to provide prolonged rescue breathing, but no more than thirty minutes of chest compressions. If there are multiple victims, institute reverse triage principles; i.e., treat seemingly dead victims first.

Therapy for increased intracranial pressure (see chapters 4 and 5) may be necessary.

For conscious patients capable of safely tolerating oral fluids, hydrate appropriately to safeguard against the rarely encountered but possible rhabdomyolysis.

Promptly investigate the hypotensive patient for major hemorrhage, spinal shock, or fluid loss from burns. Internal burns of muscles may result in extensive fluid loss, out of proportion to the external burns. Burns requiring burn-center therapy are rarely a requirement. Test vision and evaluate hearing. Tetanus immunization must be current. Evacuate all patients surviving a lightning strike for definitive medical evaluation and treatment. These patients have a potential for immediate and delayed sequelae, including neurological, renal, cardiac, and muscular dysfunction.

CHAPTER

15

Field Water Disinfection

Recommendations are considered Category 1B by the WMS Panel of Expert Reviewers.

I. GENERAL INFORMATION

All surface water carries a risk of enteric illness due to ingestion of waterborne pathogens that include bacteria, viruses, protozoan cysts, and some parasitic eggs or larvae. Risk varies with geographic location. In North America, *Giardia lamblia* is the most common microbial contaminant, but *Campylobacter jejuni,* enterotoxigenic *E. coli,* enteric viruses, and *Cryptosporidium* have caused outbreaks of illness. In developing countries, surface and tap water must be considered contaminated. Potential microorganisms include protozoa (*Entamoeba histolytica, Giardia lamblia, Cryptosporidium*), bacteria (*E. coli, Shigella, Vibrio cholerae, Salmonella, C. jejuni, V. parahaemolyticus*), viruses (hepatitis A and other enteric viruses), or helminths. Potable drinking water can be prepared by disinfecting water using one of several means.

II. METHODS OF WATER DISINFECTION

A. Heat

As in pasteurization, temperatures above 160°F (70°C) kill all enteric pathogens within thirty minutes, and 185°F (85°C) is effective within a few minutes. Thus, disinfection occurs during the time required to heat water from 140°F (60°C) to boiling temperature, so any water brought to a boil, even at high altitudes, is safe.

B. Filtration

Filtration may be used for *Giardia* and other protozoal cysts, enteric bacteria, and parasitic eggs. However, for field use, filtration alone does not adequately remove viruses, although many are removed by adhering to larger particles. The maximum effective filter pore size for *Giardia* and amoeba cysts is 5 microns. For enteric bacteria it is 0.2 to 0.5 microns, depending on filter design. *Cryptosporidium* oocysts require less than 3 microns pore size, while other parasitic eggs and larvae are removed with a 20- to 30-micron filter. Most commercial filters claim removal of *Giardia* only or *Giardia* and bacteria. Claims for viral removal should be discounted because they are not well substantiated. Some filters incorporate activated charcoal or an iodine resin. (See III.) Newer filtration systems take advantage of microtubules that provide an absolute 0.2 micron filtration size, with a rapid flow rate achieved by their massive total surface area due to the number of tubules wrapped into the filter.

C. Clarification

Clarification techniques remove suspended particulate matter and many microorganisms. They are not adequate to disinfect water reliably, but they may be used to improve clarity and remove organic matter prior to filtration or halogenation.

1. Sedimentation is the separation of large particles by gravity. Simply allow water to stand in any container for at least one hour, and then decant.

2. Coagulation, flocculation (C-F) removes smaller, suspended particles (colloids) that will not settle with simple gravity. This method works best on "cloudy" water, such as brown or green water that is loaded with organic material, as opposed to inorganic matter such as fine clay particles. Alum (aluminum sulfate) is added to water (⅛ to ¼ tsp/gal) and mixed thoroughly. Then stir or gently agitate occasionally for five minutes and allow to settle. Colloidal particles clump together and then settle by gravity or float. The clear water can be decanted, filtered, or poured through a cloth or coffee filter. The majority of microorganisms will settle with the floc, but a second disinfection step is recommended. Alum can be obtained at chemical supply stores or some grocery stores (pickling powder). If alum is not available, lime or the fine white ash from a campfire can be used.

3. Charcoal filters (purifiers) alone are not adequate for disinfection, although they improve the taste and appearance of water by absorbing chemicals.

D. Halogens

Halogens (chlorine and iodine) are effective disinfectants for viruses, bacteria, and protozoan cysts (excluding *Cryptosporidium*). Both are available in tablet or liquid form. Iodine also comes in crystalline or polymolecular resin form. In equivalent concentrations, iodine has some advantages over chlorine for field use, less reactivity with organic matter, and less sensitivity to pH.

The effectiveness of a halogen depends on its concentration, the temperature of the water, and the amount of time it is left in the water (contact time). Weaker concentrations or colder water necessitate longer contact time.

In the wilderness, the residual concentration cannot be measured, so some uncertainty results. Very high doses of halogen may be used to overcome the uncertainty, but this results in unacceptable taste. Smaller doses are effective in clean water if a prolonged contact time is used. Detection of a faint halogen color, smell, or taste indicates the presence of residual halogen in the water.

Because iodine and chlorine react with organic impurities to form a relatively inactive compound, the dose must be increased in grossly contaminated or cloudy water. Inorganic particulate matter does not react with halogens but can be removed by straining, filtering, sedimentation, or coagulation to improve taste. It is best to clarify water before treatment with halogens. Palatable surface water has a nearly neutral pH, which is optimal for effective treatment with a halogen.

Taste may be improved by several means:

■ Decrease the amount of halogen while increasing contact time.
■ Add flavored drink mix after adequate contact time.
■ Pour water through a charcoal filter after adequate contact time.
■ Use techniques that do not leave residual halogen, such as heat or filters.
■ Remove the halogen taste by using a zinc brush (see below), sodium thiosulfate, ascorbic acid (vitamin C), or hydrogen peroxide in combination with calcium hypochlorite (see below).

An alternative to iodine should be sought for pregnant women (although the amount ingested from a filter with an iodine resin is safe). Caution should be exercised if iodine is used for more than two weeks with anyone on Lithium (establish stable medication dose and confirm normal thyroid function) or with an active thyroid disease. Women older than fifty are at some risk of hypothyroidism.

III. TECHNIQUES FOR WATER DISINFECTION

A. Iodine resins

The resin releases iodine on contact that binds to microorganisms. The exact mechanism of iodine transfer to organisms is not known. Minimal iodine dissolves in water: effluent contains 0.5 to 2 ppm iodine. This dissolved iodine is not responsible for disinfection, so many filters include a charcoal resin to remove all iodine dissolved in the water after passing through the iodine resin. Some devices incorporate a 1-micron filter to remove cysts that are resistant to iodine (*Cryptosporidium*) or require longer contact times (*Giardia*). Potential problems include channeling of water through the resin, which may allow some organisms through without contacting the iodine resin.

WATER DISINFECTION TECHNIQUES AND HALOGEN DOSES[*]

Iodination techniques Added to 1 liter or quart of clear water	amount for 4 ppm	amount for 8 ppm
Iodine tabs tetraglycine hydroperiodide EDWGT (emergency drinking water germicidal tablet) Potable Aqua Globaline	$^1/_2$ tab	1 tab
2% iodine solution (tincture)	0.2 ml 5 gtts	0.4 ml 10 gtts
10% povidone-iodine solution**	0.35 ml 8 gtts	0.70 ml 16 gtts
Saturated solution: iodine crystals in water	13 ml	26 ml
Saturated solution: iodine crystals in alcohol	0.1 ml	0.2 ml
Chlorination techniques	**amount for 5 ppm**	**amount for 10 ppm**
Household bleach 5% Sodium hypochlorite	0.1 ml 2 gtts	0.2 ml 4 gtts
AquaClear Sodium dichloroisocyanurate		1 tab
AquaCure, AquaPure, Chlor-floc Chlorine plus flocculating agent		8 ppm/tab

*Measure with dropper (1drop=0.05 ml) or tuberculin syringe.
**Povidone-iodine solutions release free iodine in levels adequate for disinfection, but scant data are available.

Concentration of halogen	Contact time in minutes at various water temperatures		
	5°C/41°F	15°C/59°F	30°C/86°F
2 ppm	240	180	60
4 ppm	180	60	45
8 ppm	60	30	15

NOTE: These contact times have been extended from the usual recommendations to account for recent data that prolonged contact time is needed in very cold water to kill *Giardia* cysts.

Recommended doses are doubled for cloudy water. The optimal method is to clarify water prior to treating.

B. Chlorination-dechlorination

This technique uses very high concentrations of chlorine for disinfection, then "dechlorination" with peroxide, which forms soluble calcium chloride, a tasteless and odorless compound. Excess peroxide bubbles off as oxygen. The kit consists of chlorine crystals (calcium hypochloride) and 30 percent hydrogen peroxide in separate small Nalgene bottles. This is a very good technique for highly polluted or cloudy waters, for disinfecting large volumes, and for storing water on boats. *NOTE:* 30 percent peroxide is extremely corrosive and burns skin.

C. Flocculation-chlorination

Tablets contain both alum as a flocculent and chlorine as a disinfectant. This has the advantage of cleaning and disinfecting cloudy or foul-smelling water in a one-step process. The tablet is designed to leave 8 ppm free residual chlorine after flocculation, but 3 to 5 ppm is more common. Extend the recommended fifteen-minute contact time for added safety in cold water.

D. Dehalogenation

A small wand with brushlike zinc and copper alloy bristles is used to stir the water to dechlorinate. It is intended to be used after halogenation. Zinc catalyses an electrochemical reaction reducing hypochlorite to chloride or iodine to iodide, neither of which have taste, smell, or color. Zinc is not used up, so the life span of the product is indefinite. The device is practical only for small amounts of water at a time. Larger volumes or higher concentrations require a considerable amount of time. Very small amounts of sodium thiosulfate or ascorbic acid will accomplish the same chemical reduction, removing halogen taste. These techniques should only be used after adequate contact time.

IV. CONTROVERSIES

What is the best technique?

The best technique depends on personal preference and intended use. Use of heat may be limited by fuel supplies. If planned for a large group, halogenation or high-capacity filters work best. Two-stage techniques are more effective as water quality deteriorates.

Iodine and chlorine have similar antimicrobial activity, although there may be some advantages to iodine. Most prefer the taste of iodine over chlorine in equipotent doses, and iodine is less reactive with nitrogenous wastes in the water. However, iodine is physiologically active and may be unsafe for individuals with iodine allergies, for those with uncontrolled thyroid disease, and for prolonged use in pregnant women. Although not proven dangerous in healthy individuals, iodine use should be limited to months, not years.

Filtration is not a reliable method of removing viruses. Although viral contamination is currently unlikely in North American alpine surface water, high levels of viral contamination should be assumed in lowland rivers with towns upstream and in developing countries. In these areas, halogenation or heat should be used instead of, or in addition to, filtration.

Is **Cryptosporidium** *a sufficient risk to mandate filtration of surface water?*

Cryptosporidium is a protozoan, transmitted by the fecal-oral route, that can cause enteric illness. It produces a hardy oocyst. Waterborne outbreaks have been demonstrated, and the oocysts have been found to be widespread in surface water. Although pathogenicity is not debated, the epidemiology of infection, specifically the incidence of symptomatic infection and presence of immunity, is unclear. The problem is that the oocyst is extremely resistant to halogens.

Are waterborne pathogens a significant source of illness for wilderness and foreign travelers?

The major source of traveler's diarrhea is foodborne. However, waterborne outbreaks of most enteric pathogens have been confirmed, and the waterborne route has been shown to be a major source of giardiasis outbreaks in the United States, especially from surface water. While the risk of illness from wilderness water in North America may be small and considered negligible by some, countries without sanitation have a much higher risk due to high levels of enteric pathogens in surface water.

CHAPTER

16

Oral Fluid and Electrolyte Replacement

Recommendations are considered Category 1B by the WMS Panel of Expert Reviewers.

I. GENERAL INFORMATION

Oral rehydration/electrolyte solutions (ORS) are useful in three circumstances when fluids and electrolytes may be lost in significant amounts:

- Heavy, prolonged exercise with high-volume sweat losses
- Treatment of mild to moderate heat illness
- Illness with diarrhea and/or vomiting

Significant hemorrhage also requires fluid replacement.

A. Fluid replacement during exercise

Large fluid losses may occur during exercise in heat and at high altitudes. Sweat losses of 1 L/h are common during moderate exercise in a hot environment or at high levels of exertion in a temperate environment. The rate is individual and depends on the degree of heat acclimatization. Dehydration disposes to heat illness. In high-altitude mountaineering, the scarcity of surface water, difficulty adjusting clothing to changing levels of exertion or weather conditions, and respiratory fluid losses from hyperventilation in dry, cold air (averages 1.5 L/day for moderate exertion at 15,000 feet [4,500 meters]) commonly creates fluid needs of 7 to 8 L/day. Dehydration in this environment disposes to altitude sickness, hypothermia, frostbite, and venous thrombosis.

During exercise, frequent fluid replacement is critical. Inadequate fluid intake decreases exercise performance and increases the risk of heat illness. Too much fluid may lead to dilutional hyponatremia. For most situations, at least 300–500 ml per hour will be required. Hydration needs will be higher with extreme exertion or environment. The fluid is best consumed in volumes of approximately 200 ml at a time as this promotes emptying of the stomach. Dark urine suggests that the body is struggling to maintain normal hydration and can be used as a sign that fluid intake should be increased.

Sweat contains electrolytes: sodium (average 20 to 60 mEq/L), chloride, and small amounts of potassium. In most instances, replacement of electrolytes during sweat loss, especially during less than sixty minutes of exercise, is not necessary, so ORS have no advantage over plain water. Electrolyte needs during prolonged physical activity can usually be met by regular meals and snacks, which also provide more calories than electrolyte solutions.

In endurance events or work/exercise in a very hot environment with high sweat losses, electrolyte supplements are recommended. During exercise, a solution containing 2 to 6 percent glucose and 30 mEq/L sodium is optimal to maintain palatability. Higher glucose concentrations may delay gastric emptying and promote osmotic diarrhea, but new long-chain carbohydrates that break down to simple sugars during digestion can provide larger amounts of sugar. Excessive sodium can cause nausea. Do not ingest salt tablets directly because they can cause gastric irritation and vomiting. One or two salt tablets, however, can be dissolved in a liter of water. Commercial sports drinks contain about 6 percent glucose and 10 to 25 mEq/L of sodium. Simple solutions can be made at home. One tsp/L sugar yields a 0.35 to 0.5 percent solution, so 3 to 4 tsp sugar in a liter yields a 1 to 2 percent solution with about 50 kcal. One-half tsp NaCl (table salt) added to 1 liter of water yields about 30 mEq/L. In the wilderness, it is convenient to replace salt with snack foods during exertion. Although the teaspoon measurement method is quite variable (yielding 3.5 to 5 ml), concentrations over the resulting range are not dangerous.

B. Treatment of mild heat illness

Oral electrolyte solutions are an excellent means of treating mild to moderate forms of heat illness, such as heat syncope, heat cramps, and heat exhaustion. The patient must rest in the shade and sip fluids. Usually 1 to 2 liters of fluids similar to exercise replacement fluids are adequate. Oral fluids cannot be used for heat stroke, during altered consciousness, unless via a naso-gastric tube.

C. Replacement of enteric fluid losses

Diarrheal illness (e.g., traveler's diarrhea) is the main indication for oral electrolyte solutions. Most cases of infectious enteritis are self-limited, although antibiotics can shorten the duration of most bacterial enteric infections. The major morbidity from these infections results from dehydration, so rehydration and maintenance of fluids and electrolytes are essential. Diarrheal fluid contains more electrolytes than sweat: sodium (50 to 100 mEq/L), chloride, and significant amounts of potassium and bicarbonate. Oral replacement is feasible because the gut can absorb water and electrolytes when administered with glucose, even during severe secretory diarrhea.

The optimal composition of rehydration fluid for gastrointestinal losses is a sodium concentration between 50 and 90 mEq/L. The lower concentration may be more palatable, but the higher concentration is most effective with moderate dehydration. Maximal glucose concentration is 2 to 2.5 percent. Higher concentrations may have an osmotic effect, making diarrhea worse. Cereal-based ORS contains complex carbohydrate molecules from rice or grains that do not create an excessive osmotic load but are digested as simple glucose. At least 20 mEq/L of potassium is necessary, and 30 mEq/L of bicarbonate is optimal.

The World Health Organization (WHO) has developed electrolyte salts specifically for diarrheal illness that contain 90 mEq of sodium, 20 mEq of potassium, 80 mEq of chloride, 30 mEq of bicarbonate or trisodium citrate, and 111 mmol (2 percent) of glucose, which must be mixed with 1 liter of disinfected water. Packets of these oral rehydration salts are distributed throughout the world by WHO and UNICEF, commonly under the name Oralyte. More expensive premixed solutions are available, but they are not practical for wilderness or foreign travel. Sports drinks and other "clear liquids" contain insufficient sodium and potassium and excessive glucose for treatment of diarrheal-induced dehydration, but they are better than plain water.

If premeasured salts are not available, a substitute recommended by the Centers for Disease Control and Prevention (CDC) consists of alternating glasses of the following two fluids:

■ Glass 1: 8 oz (250 ml) fruit juice (such as apple, orange, or lemon), ½ tsp honey or corn syrup, and 1 pinch salt
■ Glass 2: 8 oz (250 ml) water (boiled or treated) and ¼ tsp baking soda
These ingredients, however, may not be available to remote travelers.

Plain salt and sugar solutions, similar to those used for heat/exercise replacement, can be used for mild dehydration, but they are not adequate for serious dehydration or replacement of continuing high losses. For mild dehydration, partial maintenance, or supplementation, or where nothing else is available, rice water, fruit juice, coconut milk, or diluted cola drinks may suffice.

II. GUIDELINES FOR FLUID REPLACEMENT

Achieve replacement of estimated fluid deficit in about four hours by giving 50 ml/kg body weight for mild dehydration and 100 ml/kg for moderate dehydration. This means that for mild dehydration, an adult should drink 250 ml of oral rehydration solution every thirty minutes for the first four to six hours. Children should drink 200 to 250 ml/hour. In addition, they may drink water as desired. Give infants younger than three months a 100 ml dose each hour, with every third dose replaced by plain water. Ingestion of frequent, small amounts, rather than rapid ingestion, minimizes vomiting. Fluid deficit is replaced within twelve hours in 90 percent of patients. Determine maintenance fluids by estimating or measuring stool losses plus normal maintenance requirements. Since this is not often possible in the field, give 10 to 15 ml/kg body weight/diarrheal stool.

At least 90 percent of patients during diarrhea epidemics can be successfully rehydrated using only ORS. Failure of ORS occurs when stool losses exceed oral intake. Vomiting, unless frequent and protracted, does not preclude rehydration with oral solutions. Fluids may be administered by nasogastric tube when the patient is unable or unwilling to drink adequate fluids. Intravenous fluids can be reserved for the initial hydration of patients with shock, obtundation, seizures, or intractable vomiting. When IV fluids are necessary, ORS usually can be initiated within four hours and exclusively used within twenty-four hours.

III. CONTROVERSIES

Does ORS cause hypernatremia in patients without cholera?
Many physicians in developed countries avoid ORS because of an unsubstantiated concern for hypernatremia in small children. This concern has led to lower sodium concentrations (50 to 75 mEq/L) in commercial ORS sold in the United States and recommendations to use the higher concentration only for initial rehydration, then lower concentrations for maintenance. This complexity can be avoided if plain water or formula is alternated with ORS in the maintenance phase of treatment.

Are electrolyte-replacement drinks necessary for wilderness activities?
Cases of severe hyponatremia in endurance athletes and recreational hikers in hot climates have been reported, and they were probably caused by "water intoxication." As sweat losses increase with environmental heat stress and prolonged exercise, electrolyte replacement becomes more important. Most wilderness sports, such as hiking, climbing, or skiing, offer frequent opportunities to rest and ingest food and fluids. If snack foods are eaten regularly, plain water will be safe for fluid replacement. Unfortunately, many hikers favor snack foods that are high in carbohydrates and fats (such as candy) but low in sodium. Some individuals, noting the edema present in their hands and feet associated with heat or altitude exposure, attempt to restrict their sodium intake. The development of heat exhaustion causes nausea, preventing food intake. If frequent snack and meal breaks are not planned, recommend electrolyte replacement fluids for sustained wilderness activities in hot climates.

17

Botanical Encounters

Recommendations are considered Category 1B, except where indicated 1A, by the WMS Panel of Expert Reviewers.

I. GENERAL INFORMATION

The majority of botanical problems in humans are due to contact, but some are due to ingestion, mostly of fungi. Treatment in the field depends on the nature and severity of the problem. Many contact episodes can be treated on the spot. Virtually all contacts by ingestion require urgent evacuation.

II. PLANT-INDUCED DERMATITIS

Most injuries result from simple mechanical or chemical trauma, sensitization to allergens, or a photochemical response. Dermal reactions may be immunologic, non-immunologic, or both. Injuries may be further complicated by secondary infections, *id* reactions, and further damage by excoriation or improper treatment. Identification of the offending plant is important to both treatment and future avoidance.

A. Mechanical injury and treatment

Many plants possess spines, thorns, bristles, barbs, and sharp serrated edges, contact with which can cause punctures or lacerations that often contain embedded plant material. Other plants contain specialized structures to deliver irritants that cause both mechanical and chemical injury. Numerous spines, thorns, and fine hairs, called glochids, in the cactus genus *Opuntia* can cause aseptic granulomatous lesions resembling scabies.

Follow basic wound-care principles when treating punctures and lacerations. Clean all wounds and remove any foreign material. Apply, then carefully remove, glue or tape to extract fine foreign bodies, though tape stripping was associated with increased cactus spine persistence and more inflammation in at least one experimental study (Category 1A) (reference: Martinez, T. T., M. Jerome, R. C. Barry, and J. G. Xander. 1987. Removal of cactus spines from the skin. A comparative evaluation of several methods. *Am J Dis Child* 14:1,291–92). Applying a topical steroid after spine removal may decrease inflammation.

Deeply embedded material must be excised to avoid serious complications such as osteoblastic and osteolytic changes in bone, synovitis in joints, and localized or generalized infections. If removal is not possible in a remote location, the victim must be transported for definitive care. Provide pain control as necessary, and if definitive care cannot be reached within two to three days, initiate antibiotic prophylaxis as soon as possible to reduce the chance of infection. Most infections will be caused by dermatologic organisms and are usually well covered by first-generation cephalosporins. Augmented penicillins, fluoroquinolones, and macrolide antibiotics are alternatives.

If the foreign body can be removed, antibiotic treatment should be reserved for secondary infections. Tetanus prophylaxis is required for these injuries.

Many plants contain irritants that cause reactions through their chemical or physical properties. For example, members of the family Araceae (e.g., *Dieffenbachia* or dumbcane) possess bundles of needlelike calcium oxalate crystals in their cells (raphides) that cause intense pain and itching through their microinvasive properties. Often children learn this through an unfortunate tasting experiment. These substances affect most people and are not dependent upon an individual being "allergic" to the offending agent. The reaction generally happens within seconds to minutes of the exposure, compared to "allergic" reactions that usually develop twenty to thirty minutes after contact. The two cannot be differentiated by inspection alone. Treatment consists of general cleaning with cool compresses for comfort and analgesics as necessary. Most reactions are self-limited but can be quite painful for twelve to twenty-four hours. Intense itching can be relieved with antihistamines.

Contaminated eyes should be copiously irrigated. A cycloplegic such as scopolamine 0.25 percent drops (see chapter 9) may greatly relieve pain along with the use of artificial tears. Patching is not helpful unless a foreign body cannot be removed.

B. Chemical injury and treatment

1. Allergic dermatitis

This phenomenon occurs after previous sensitization to some allergen. These agents are usually in the form of a hapten that combines with skin proteins to form an antigen. This is a cellular (type IV) reaction mediated by t-lymphocytes. In those individuals who tend to be atopic, the reaction can be eczematous.

In the United States the family Anacardiaceae, containing poison ivy (*Toxicodendron radicans*) and poison oak (*T. diversilobum*), causes more dermatitis than any other plant or household or industrial chemical. The offending agents here are various catechols. The severity of reaction to this family depends on the size and thickness of the cornified skin exposed and the dose of toxin received. Following contact, a cutaneous response occurs in twelve to twenty-four hours. This latent period can be helpful in determining the mechanism of reaction. Initially an area of erythema develops, usually with some edema. During the next twenty-four hours vesicles or bullae develop containing a nonallergic serous fluid that does not spread the dermatitis, contrary to popular belief. Exudation may be marked, and itching is intense. After several days crusting develops, and resolution occurs in ten to fourteen days, barring complications. Previously affected sites distant from the currently affected area may flare as well.

Cutaneous penetration takes about ten minutes. Therefore if exposure is immediately recognized, prompt washing may reduce the severity or prevent a reaction. Washing with water is recommended, but avoid soaps as they remove protective oils from the skin. Apply organic solvents such as alcohol carefully to avoid spreading the agent. Both topical and oral steroids are maximally effective during this period. Generally "dose-packs" are inadequate in both dose and duration, often leading to "rebound" dermatitis. Prednisone should be started with an oral dose of 0.75–1 mg/kg a day (usually 60–80 mg) for fourteen days, and then tapered by 10 mg every other day to prevent recurrence.

Avoidance of the plant is the best policy. Meticulously wash any clothing that comes into contact with the plant resin. Carefully clean exposed tools and backpacks with alcohol.

Numerous other plants can also cause reactions. It is vital to remember that some individuals may have an anaphylactic reaction to a dermal exposure. Should this occur, the first-line treatment is epinephrine (1:1000) 0.2–0.5 ml SQ or IM.

2. Contact urticaria

This reaction may be immunologic or nonimmunologic. It is characterized by a central irregularly raised wheal that is mildly blanched, surrounded by an irregular more erythematous flare. The process is caused by the release of histamines and other vasoactive agents. The reaction produces a sensation ranging from mildly itchy to intensely painful, such as those reactions caused by the Urticaceae (nettle) family. Occasionally an ipsilateral self-limiting lymphadenopathy can develop. Generally, a good cleansing of the area is all that is necessary as this process is self-limited. Administer pain and itch medication.

3. Photodermatitis

Some plant species contain psoralens that sensitize the skin to ultraviolet light. This is a phototoxic reaction—an exaggerated sunburnlike reaction. With sun exposure, more severe, even blistering burns can occur. Areas exposed need to be protected from the sun for approximately two weeks. Treatment is the same as for any sunburn. Cool compresses and administration of nonsteroidal anti-inflammatories such as ibuprofen or aspirin can be helpful.

III. PLANT INGESTIONS

Between 1994 and 1999, one million people in the United States ingested potentially dangerous plants: only twenty-seven died, and major morbidity was rare. While the majority of ingested toxins were from fungi (mushrooms), there are numerous deadly toxins, such as ricin and abrin from *Ricinus* and *Abru,* cicutoxin from *Cicuta douglasii* (water hemlock), gyratoxins from the Rhododendron family, aconitine from the genus *Acontium* (wolfsbane and monkshood) and numerous alkaloids, which all tend to present with GI symptoms. Toxicity is low with inadvertent exposures but can be fatal after a large dose, as often happens with a case of mistaken identity, "folk" remedies, and ritualistic ingestions. Later, more serious symptoms can develop with deadly consequences.

A. Diagnosis

A presumptive diagnosis can be made based upon the history and early presenting signs and symptoms. To plan treatment, every effort should be made to note the overall shape of the tree or shrub and to collect any available flowers, fruits, and foliage. Several highly toxic or fatal species look almost identical to other harmless and even delicious plants. Toxicities within and among species can vary greatly depending upon location, and a poor correlation exists between taxonomy and toxicity. Consequently, clinical judgment and reevaluation of the victim are of the utmost importance.

B. Mushroom ingestions

If mushroom poisoning is suspected, urgently evacuate to definitive medical care. Initiate seizure precautions. Vomiting is a common result of mushroom poisoning. A late onset of gastric cramping and vomiting may be a more serious prognostic indicator than early onset of symptoms. Almost *none* of the mushroom toxins are changed by heat or drying. Therefore, cooking the plants does not remove the danger, and toxicity can occur from inhalation of mushroom fumes as well as from ingestion.

C. Treatment

Treatment in the field is, of necessity, limited because the diagnosis may be uncertain and the appropriate therapeutic agents—such as activated charcoal—are rarely, if ever, included in a first-aid kit. It should be noted that while activated charcoal is widely used as first-line treatment, there are surprisingly no good randomized double-blinded studies to support it as the standard of care for toxin ingestion. (References: Bradberry, S. M., and J. A. Vale. 1995. Multiple-dose activated charcoal: A review of relevant clinical studies. *J Toxicol Clin Toxicol* 33:407–16. Manoguerra, A. S. 1997. Gastrointestinal decontamination after poisoning. Where is the science? *Crit Care Clin* 13:709–25.)

If vomiting can be induced within the first few minutes after ingestion, in an alert patient, some benefit may be achieved. The induction of vomiting after thirty minutes is of no benefit.

All victims of known, or suspected, toxic ingestion should be evacuated as rapidly as possible. If the victim develops seizures, benzodiazepines may be helpful for their control. An unconscious patient must be checked frequently to maintain and protect the airway, which may become compromised by excessive salivation or secretions.

IV. CONTROVERSIES

Is vomiting a beneficial reflex? Should syrup of ipecac be administered in the treatment of poisoning?

A position statement by the American Academy of Clinical Toxicology and the European Association of Poisons Centres and Clinical Toxicologists (1997) indicates that there was insufficient data to support or exclude ipecac administration soon after poison ingestion. This position statement advises against the routine use of syrup of ipecac in the management of poisoned patients.

CHAPTER

18

Marine Envenomations and Poisonings

Recommendations are considered Category 1B by the WMS Panel of Expert Reviewers.

I. GENERAL INFORMATION

Marine creatures may cause illness both by injection (envenomation) and ingestion (poisoning) of the multitude of toxins they elaborate. There is a broad range of species involved, and these are widely distributed. In general, tropical and subtropical environments are the highest risk areas. Many of the venoms and toxins involved are still poorly characterized, yet there are recognizable themes across species in patterns of envenomation and management.

II. GUIDELINES FOR PREVENTION

Prevention of marine envenomations and poisonings requires local knowledge. In general, common sense is required. Few marine creatures are aggressive unless disturbed. Stout footwear is an obvious precaution when walking through shallows, especially coral or rocks. Do not handle marine creatures—observe them from a distance. During high-risk periods, wear "stinger suits" to minimize the risk of jellyfish envenomation and, where possible, swim at safe beaches or in protected enclosures. Know which species of fish and seafood can be safely eaten at any given time. Perhaps most importantly, know the risks of your local environment. Know the appropriate first aid and be aware of the definitive care of each condition.

III. GUIDELINES FOR ASSESSMENT AND TREATMENT

Other than attention to the ABCs, care of the victim of a marine envenomation or poisoning may include: prevention of further envenomation, venom neutralization, pain relief, specific antivenoms, specific adjunctive drug therapy, and surgical wound care.

A. Jellyfish

This group covers an enormous range of genus and species. They share a common means of envenomation through thousands of tiny stinging capsules (nematocysts), which come into contact with exposed flesh that passes through their trailing tentacles. Some of the medically more important include the box jellyfish (*Chironex*), man-o-war, and the irukandji. Immediate and often severe local pain is the rule with jellyfish stings. Most jellyfish will also cause a prominent skin rash. The most severe envenomations (especially those of the box jellyfish) may lead to respiratory failure and cardiovascular collapse.

For all types of box jellyfish stings, vinegar (4–6 percent acetic acid) splashed liberally over the areas where stingers are adherent has been shown to reliably inhibit nematocyst discharge and inactivate remaining undischarged nematocysts. This therapy is not proven to be effective or harmful in other jellyfish envenomations. Once inactivated, remaining stingers should be plucked off with gloved fingers or forceps. Dried nematocysts may be reactivated by water exposure, so stingers should be physically removed and not washed off. Pressure immobilization bandaging as used in elapid snakebites may be useful first aid, especially in box jellyfish envenomation.

B. Venomous fish stings

Many fish and rays possess sharp stinging spines capable of causing local trauma and, through injection of venom, intense local pain. Deaths have been associated with many species either due to direct local trauma or to the effects of envenomation. Secondary local infection and local tissue damage is often described. Retained local foreign bodies are common.

Pain relief in these cases is usually obtained by immersion of the affected area in hot water. Whether this technique works by venom neutralization or other local effects is uncertain. Care must be taken to test the hot water beforehand. The water should be as hot as can be comfortably tolerated (104–110°F, 40–43°C), but not so hot as to cause burns, particularly if the area is anaesthetized. Narcotic analgesia or injected local anesthesia may be required to ensure pain control. Antivenom, which is injected intramuscularly, is available and is effective against stonefish. Any venomous fish sting requires careful wound examination and even surgical care to ensure that retained foreign bodies are avoided.

C. Sea snakes

Bites from these creatures are a common cause of envenomation on a world-wide scale, especially in the Indo-Pacific regions. Sea snakes are generally nonaggressive and will only attack if provoked or interfered with. The effects of their venom, clinical manifestations, and treatment are the same as for other elapid snakes (see chapter 20). In particular, pressure-immobilization bandaging and rapid transfer to a medical facility for specific antivenom therapy may be lifesaving.

D. Mollusk envenomations

The two most notable are coneshells and blue ring octopus, both of which may inject rapid acting neurotoxins. These produce a progressive paralysis that has been associated with a number of deaths. The key to management is recognition and support of ventilation (using mouth-to-mouth in the field if required). Pressure-immobilization bandaging may help to limit venom spread and the onset of toxic effects (see chapter 20).

E. Marine poison ingestions

On a worldwide scale, these are likely to be the single largest cause of mortality associated with encounters with marine creatures. Poisoning with tetrodotoxin occurs from eating the flesh of incorrectly prepared pufferfish ("fugu"). Although slower in onset, the manifestations and required management will be similar to that seen with blue ring octopus envenomation. Again, the key lifesaving intervention is artificial support of ventilation.

Paralytic shellfish poisoning is due to ingestion of mollusks that have themselves ingested and concentrated the poison saxitoxin that is produced by microscopic dinoflagellates. This toxin produces a rapid onset of paralysis that is managed in the same way as pufferfish poisoning.

Cigautera poisoning occurs from eating fish that have concentrated toxins passed up the food chain from dinoflagellates. The illness is particularly common in parts of the South Pacific and West Indies. Specific species of fish are recognized as the common causes in specific geographic locations, with the onset being one to twenty-four hours after the fish ingestion. Symptoms vary but commonly include: diarrhea, nausea, abdominal pain, muscle aches, numbness or burning of the skin, irritability, and loss of balance. The gastrointestinal symptoms usually only last a day or two, while the neurological symptoms may persist for weeks. Symptoms will be worsened by alcohol. The best treatment is prevention, by avoiding eating fish that are likely to be affected.

19

Wild Land-Animal Attacks

Recommendations are considered Category 1B by the WMS Panel of Expert Reviewers.

I. GENERAL INFORMATION

Although few truly large and wild animals remain in the contiguous United States, injuries from attacks by alligators, bison, bears, and cougars (mountain lions) occur annually. In Alaska and overseas, wild-animal attacks are a more significant cause of morbidity and mortality. Many of these involve predation by the big cats or by bears, but other species such as elephant, rhinoceros, wild pig, or hippopotamus also attack humans.

Injuries from large wild-animal attack result from a variety of mechanisms, including biting, clawing, chewing, goring, tossing, or trampling. As a result, the victim often sustains major trauma far beyond a simple bite, involving multiple organ systems and locations. Wounds are frequently contaminated with oral or soil pathogens.

Rabies should be considered a possibility after a bite or mucous membrane contact with any suspicious animal (see IV).

A. Wild cats

Wild cats spring from behind to attack the neck of their prey, sometimes crushing the trachea or sharply hyperextending the neck to fracture the cervical spine and transect the spinal cord and great vessels with their teeth.

B. Horned animals

Goring injuries from animals such as bull, American buffalo, bison, elephant, or rhinoceros produce deep puncture wounds. These may rip along fascial planes or penetrate deeply, and evisceration is not uncommon. Trampling or tossing by these animals also results in blunt trauma to the victim.

C. Bears

Bears of all types claw, bite, crush, and tear their victims. Attacks are often aimed preferentially at the head, with extensive facial injuries and scalping. Chewing on extremities is also frequently described.

D. Alligators/crocodiles

These animals tend to drown their victims before feeding on them. Victims who escape incur bite/puncture wounds that invariably become infected without treatment.

II. PREVENTION

For all wild-animal attacks, prevention can be summarized as "Don't get too close—stay out of the way." Approaching animals too closely while photographing is particularly risky. Alertness and awareness of the animal habitat during wilderness travel will prevent many encounters. Travel and camp using techniques to avoid close contact with wild animals; e.g., avoid obvious large-animal paths, avoid areas dotted with fresh scat, do not sleep with food or other aromatic substances, store food and scented objects in portable or on-site bear canisters, or hang food well above the ground and away from tents. There is safety in numbers. Group travel, therefore, is safer than solo travel.

General recommendations in case of an attack or encounter include attempting to remove the perceived threat to the animal—i.e., you. In an unanticipated encounter, slowly and quietly back away. Running away will often elicit a predatory response. "Playing dead" by dropping to the ground, rolling into a knee-to-chest ball, and covering your head and face with your arms is advised in a sudden grizzly encounter. These maneuvers all "remove the threat."

If an attack is unprovoked, with human seen as prey, aggressively fighting back is recommended. Behavior such as advancing rather than fleeing, making loud noises, or waving arms to appear larger and more threatening may forestall an attack. Vigorous resistance with physical fighting, including striking the attacking animal with fists or any object or weapon, has been effective in repelling attacks by cougars, lions, tigers, brown and black bears, and even crocodiles. Cayenne pepper spray may be useful if approached by a bear. Many people carry firearms in "bear country." Both pepper spray and firearms may provide a false sense of security as both must be used correctly by persons trained in their use to be effective.

Avoidance is best. Common sense dictates care in traveling, camping, food storage, cooking, and sleeping. Preparation with a plan of action in case of an attack is strongly advised.

III. GUIDELINES FOR ASSESSMENT AND TREATMENT

Scene safety is an initial consideration for rescuers: Is the animal gone or liable to attack again? Do not spend time tracking the attacking animal unless adequate assistance to the victim is simultaneously available and rescuers are experienced and competent in such activity.

Attend to the ABCs as always. Airway management may be complicated with head, facial, neck, or chest injuries. Assume all victims of large wild-animal attacks have sustained multiple traumas. Beyond the obvious bite, claw, or goring wounds, the victim needs assessment for fractures, neurovascular damage, and internal head, chest, and abdominal injury. Try to determine the mechanisms of injury. Soft-tissue damage far beyond the obvious may result from trampling, butting, or tossing with ground impact. Bites regularly penetrate more deeply than apparent. Recognize the factor of psychological trauma, even in the field.

Wound cleaning is the single most important step in preventing infection; its importance cannot be overemphasized (see chapter 6). Splint large open wounds and fractures (see chapter 8). Cover abdominal eviscerations and eye injuries with a moist, clean dressing—and evacuate rapidly.

Vigorously irrigate animal bites with water safe to drink, then scrub with soap and water, followed by a sixty- to ninety-second rinse with a 1 percent concentration of povidone-iodine or 0.5 percent chlorhexidine gluconate, if available. Except where necessary to control hemorrhage or to allow extrication, never close or tightly approximate an animal bite wound in the wilderness. Devitalized, necrotic tissue from bite and crush injuries requires debridement. Many of these injuries are contaminated; the decision to close wounds after thorough irrigation and debridement should consider the risk of the patient (higher risk for immune-compromised patients) and of the wound (higher risk if deep punctures, contaminated with oral flora, in the hand or poorly vascularized tissues). High-risk wound and/or high-risk patients should receive prophylactic antibiotics such as amoxicillin-clavulanate, a second- or third-generation cephalosporin, a quinolone, a penicillinase-resistant penicillin, or a tetracycline antibiotic (erythromycin is not an acceptable alternative). Wild cats, like their domestic counterparts, inflict bite wounds contaminated with *Pasteurella multocida,* and antibiotic selection should include coverage for this pathogen. Update tetanus immunization as these injuries are high-risk wounds for tetanus.

IV. RABIES

A rabies exposure consists of a bite, contamination of an open wound or abrasion with saliva, or contact with any mucous membrane by saliva from an infected animal. However, in the United States, because rabies is universally lethal in humans, postexposure prophylaxis currently is often given following any contact—sometimes just close proximity—with a rabid animal. The possibility of rabies should be considered following a bite by a previously vaccinated dog or cat if the attack was unprovoked—a bite is not considered provoked if an attempt were being made to feed, pet, run by, or capture the animal—or if the animal was acting unnaturally prior to the bite.

Bites by livestock (cattle, sheep, horses) have the potential to cause rabies, although they almost never do in the United States. Consultation with a veterinarian following a bite appears advisable. Rodents and lagomorphs almost never transmit rabies to humans even though these animals, like all mammals, are susceptible to rabies. Mice and rats are used for laboratory studies.

The CDC advises that anyone bitten by any wild animal should receive rabies postexposure prophylaxis unless the animal is captured and examined for rabies.

Since 1980 all but four of the approximately thirty human rabies infections acquired in the United States have come from bats. Current recommendations to avoid bat rabies are:

■ Dwellings should be "bat-proofed."
■ Any skin contact with bats should be assiduously avoided.
■ Any person who has contact with a bat, regardless of whether a bite is thought to have occurred, should receive postexposure prophylaxis unless the bat can be examined for rabies.
■ Any person who has slept in a room in which a bat is found, particularly a child, should receive postexposure prophylaxis unless the bat is caught and examined for rabies.

Rabies therapy is a race to produce immunity before clinical signs of infection appear. Postexposure therapy consists of:

■ Thorough cleansing of the wound to reduce the viral inoculum
■ Administration of rabies immune globulin, as much as possible around the wound
■ Administration of a cell-culture rabies vaccine (in the deltoid muscle only) on days 0, 3, 7, 14, and 28

All three elements are equally essential; deaths have occurred when any one was neglected.

Travelers to regions where rabies is prevalent, which is most of the developing world, should consider preexposure vaccination. Such prior immunization eliminates the need for immune globulin following exposure, which is of major significance because only about one-third of the immune globulin needed for postexposure therapy is now being produced worldwide.

V. GUIDELINES FOR EVACUATION

Victims of large wild-animal attack, even with stable vital signs, usually require rapid evacuation from the field for surgical wound treatment, as well as multiple trauma evaluation with diagnostic studies such as X-ray or computed tomography. Lesser wounds or bites may require evacuation for antibiotic treatment, rabies prophylaxis, cosmetic closure, or wound exploration and cleaning.

If rescue and evacuation will require days versus hours, close observation of vital signs; daily wound care with additional field irrigation, cleaning, debridement, and dressing change as needed; and antibiotic administration is advised.

20

Reptile Envenomations

Recommendations are considered Category 1B, except where indicated 1A, by the WMS Panel of Expert Reviewers.

I. GENERAL INFORMATION

There are approximately 300,000 human snakebites worldwide each year from 2,700 known species. In the United States it is estimated that there are 45,000 bites of humans, with 8,000 envenomations and five to twelve deaths per year. The incidence of bites and fatality rates may be much higher in other parts of the world. In general, fatalities are more frequent where the snakes are more venomous (e.g., Australia) or where lay knowledge regarding venomous bites and access to medical care is lacking (e.g., parts of Asia and Africa). Venomous snakes can be broadly divided into Crotalidae (pit vipers—including rattlesnakes, cottonmouths, and copperheads) and the family Elapidae (which includes coral snakes and all venomous Australian snakes). There are about 3,000 known species of lizards, but only members of the family Helodermatidae (including Gila monsters) are considered venomous. They are found exclusively in the southwestern United States and Mexico. Lizards rarely cause human fatalities. Fatalities from U.S. crotalid envenomation are not common, but complications may be severe.

A. Pit vipers

Crotalids have a triangular head, catlike vertical pupils, hinged fangs, and a heat-sensitive "pit" on each side of the head between the tip of the nose and the eye. Rattlesnakes have a variable number of rattles depending upon age and number of molts. They sometimes strike without rattling. About 60 percent of this country's venomous bites are attributed to rattlesnakes. Cottonmouths (water moccasins) and copperheads are the other two commonly encountered North American pit vipers. Copperhead and cottonmouth venoms are quite similar and are weaker than most rattlesnake venoms. Bites by cottonmouths tend to be more serious than copperhead bites because it is a bigger snake.

B. Elapidae

These species are widely distributed, most particularly in the Southern Hemisphere. They are notable for bites that cause profound systemic effects such as neuromuscular paralysis and coagulopathy and myonecrosis, but often with minimal local effects. Identification of species even by trained observers is notoriously difficult and is not to be used to guide therapy. The several species of coral snakes are brightly colored, with black noses and alternating red-yellow-red-black bands around their bodies (remember "red on yellow can kill a fellow"). They have relatively small mouths with fixed fangs. From southern Mexico through tropical South America the rules for distinguishing coral snakes are highly unreliable. Unless you are a knowledgeable herpetologist, it is best not to pick up colorful snakes in tropical America.

C. Gila monsters

These lizards are not large, seldom reaching 20 inches in length. They have blunt heads, beady eyes, and powerful digging claws on short legs. They are shy and appear sluggish but are capable of swift, determined lunges when threatened or handled.

II. PREVENTION

Wilderness travelers are rarely bitten by venomous reptiles. Avoid reptile bites by:

■ Staying away from infested areas
■ Not hiking during times of peak reptile activity (usually at night)
■ Watching clearly where one steps
■ Never reaching into concealed areas (gathering firewood at night, for example)
■ Checking bedding, clothing, and footwear before use
■ Never handling a venomous reptile, even if it is presumed dead (reflex allows some snakes to strike even after death)

The chance of envenomation from a strike can be minimized by wearing high leather boots and long pants. Envenomation is more apt to occur in persons who are intoxicated and in young children. It is helpful to know the distribution, markings, and characteristics of venomous reptiles in intended areas of wilderness travel.

III. GUIDELINES FOR ASSESSMENT AND TREATMENT

A. Pit vipers

As many as 20 to 30 percent of crotalid bites cause no envenomation. Most, but not all, crotalid envenomations result in immediate pain at the bite site and a rapid onset (within ten to fifteen minutes) of swelling and ecchymosis. Rarely, signs of envenomation are delayed for several hours. Typical paired fang wounds are not always present. A single puncture or a scratch may be the only mark, and the degree of envenomation does not correlate with the size, quality, and number of fang marks.

Assessment of envenomation by a pit viper is the first step in managing a bite in the field. Mark the advancing border of edema and sequentially measure and mark the circumference at the site and at least one location above the bite to detect spreading edema. Reassess these measurements every fifteen minutes. Gently cleanse the area. Apply a sterile or clean dressing. The basic tenet is to provide calm, rapid transport to a medical facility. For an extremity bite, splint the limb. Do not use pressure dressings, tourniquets, applications of cold, electric shocks, or incisions of the bite site, as these techniques have no known efficacy. Lymphatic constricting bands (barely indenting the skin) are advocated by some, although their use has not been proven to have any definite advantage in pit viper envenomations.

Encourage the patient to rest and stay calm. Keep the extremity at heart level or lower. Walking out should not be attempted unless no other evacuation means is available. Walking out, however, is imperative if the patient is alone. Severe manifestations of poisoning may not occur for several hours, so travel is possible in most cases.

For those with the skill and equipment, use of oxygen is recommended, as is one large-bore (16 g or larger) IV in an unaffected limb. Start at least two large-bore IVs in a patient presenting with shock. Administer either normal saline or Ringer's lactate solution (LR) to support systolic blood pressure above 90 mmHg. Intubation or vasopressors are rarely necessary in crotalid envenomations. Field use of intravenous antivenin is not recommended.

B. Elapidae

Immediate local symptoms and signs from these bites may be minimal. The degree and rapidity of the onset of systemic symptoms will vary according to the species, bite site, and effectiveness of the bite. Systemic symptoms such as nausea, vomiting, sweating, myalgias, and general malaise are common. Signs of paralysis, such as generalized weakness, blurred vision, and respiratory difficulties, may become obvious. There may be no signs of overwhelming coagulopathy until a catastrophe such as an intracerebral bleed occurs. In all cases of suspected bite, assume envenomation and treat accordingly. There is strong evidence that in elapid bites, appropriate first aid may be lifesaving (Category 1A) (reference: Suthurland, S. K., A. R. Coulter, and R. D. Harris. 1979. Rationalisation of first-aid measures for elapid snakebite. *Lancet* 1:183–86). A bandage applied at a similar tension to that for a sprained ankle should commence at the bite site and extend along the length of the limb and back again to the bite. Splint the limb and keep the patient still. The patient must not self-evacuate under any circumstances as activity will enhance movement of the venom centrally. With well-conducted first aid, venom will be trapped and broken down locally, and the risk of life-threatening envenomation will be minimized. With the acknowledged problems in elapid species identification and of antivenom storage, the field use of antivenom is not recommended.

C. Gila monsters

Gila monsters have no injection mechanism for their venom, but they have very powerful jaws, and they chew and tear at their victims, drooling venom and producing a substantial amount of pain. Envenomation produces pain, swelling, vomiting, increased heart rate, vertigo, shortness of breath, and loss of consciousness. Follow the recommendations for pit viper envenomation. Fatal Gila monster encounters are extremely rare.

CHAPTER

21

Arthropod Envenomations

Recommendations are considered Category 1A, except where indicated 2, by the WMS Panel of Expert Reviewers.

I. GENERAL INFORMATION

In the United States, arthropods (invertebrates with jointed legs and segmented bodies) cause more deaths by envenomation than reptiles. Hymenoptera (bees, wasps, etc.), the Arachnida (spiders and scorpions), and Chilopoda (centipedes) cause the most significant envenomations.

Neither *Latrodectus* (North American black widow, Australian red-back, New Zealand kati, South African knoppie) nor *Loxosceles* (brown recluse) are aggressive toward humans. These spiders live in crevices under ground cover, trash piles, barns, porches, and outside toilets. Prevention includes inspection, clearing, and care, especially around these areas. Nearly half of all bites could be prevented if toilets and clothing were inspected prior to use. The Northwest "Hobo" spider (*Tegenaria agrestis*) has systemic and local reactions similar to mild cases of loxoscelism (reference: Vest, D. K., L. V. Boyer, J. T. McNally, and G. J. Binford. 2001. Spider bites. In *Wilderness medicine,* 4th ed., P. S. Auerbach, 829. St. Louis, Mo.: Mosby).

II. GUIDELINES FOR ASSESSMENT AND TREATMENT

A. Stinging insects

The most common insect stings are from the Hymenoptera. Although it takes about 300 to 500 stings to make a lethal dose of the complex venom, hypersensitivity, which occurs in approximately 1 percent of the general public, may result in a life-threatening anaphylactic reaction from a solitary sting. This is more common in adults than in children.

The Hymenoptera comprise four families: honeybees, which account for the most stings and leave the stinger attached to their victims; bumblebees; hornets, yellow jackets, and wasps; and fire ants, whose alkaloid venom results in a sterile, burning, vesicular lesion.

Nearly all Hymenoptera stings result in local pain, swelling, and redness. The honeybee stinger should be removed as soon as possible by the most expedient means to prevent the injection of still more venom. The site may be treated locally with gentle cleansing, application of cold, elevation, and immobilization. Calm the patient. Common remedies, such as applying a slurry of baking soda or meat tenderizer, often reduce pain. Commercial "sting sticks" containing a topical anesthetic such as xylocaine may be used. Oral aspirin or ibuprofen usually helps control pain. The use of a noninvasive suction cup, the Sawyer Extractor, helps alleviate pain and is effective in removing a portion of the venom if applied within three minutes (Category 2).

Patients with serious allergic reactions have pruritis, hives, angioedema, and early upper-airway obstruction with respiratory distress. For these individuals, apply a light constrictive band (not a tourniquet) proximal to the site. Oral antihistamines (such as diphenhydramine) may be helpful. If the patient is carrying injectable epinephrine, administer it. Arrange for evacuation as soon as possible. Maintaining ABCs may be extremely difficult without advanced knowledge and equipment.

If any signs of anaphylactic reaction are identified, rescuers carrying epinephrine should administer the drug IM (0.3 to 0.5 mg for an adult, 0.01 mg/kg up to the adult maximum for a child) or via preloaded syringes as often as necessary, depending on the patient's status.

Local infiltration with epinephrine 1:1000 (0.1–0.3 mL) near the sting site helps impede systemic absorption of venom. (References: Holgate, S. T., and M. K. Church. 1993. *Allergy,* 27, 1–27 and 29. New York: Raven Press. Marquardt, D. L., and S. I. Wasserman. 1993. Anaphylaxis. In *Allergy: Principles and practice,* Vol. II, 4th ed., ed. E. Middleton, C. E. Reed, E. F. Eliss, et al, 1,511–21. St. Louis, Mo.: Mosby. Shatz, G. S. 1992. Anaphylaxis. In *Allergy theory and practice,* 2nd ed., ed. P. E. Korenblot and H. J. Wedner, 229–41. Philadelphia: W. B. Saunders.)

B. Spider bites

There are approximately 100,000 species of spiders worldwide, with a density of up to two million spiders per acre in some areas. In the United States, the most significant venomous spiders are the black widow (*Latrodectus mactans*) and the fiddleback, also known as the brown recluse (*Loxosceles reclusa*).

The venoms of these spiders are potent toxins with numerous antigenic components capable of causing either a systemic manifestation or a local venom reaction.

1. Black widow

"Black widow" is itself a misnomer because only three of the five species of widow spider (family Therdiidae) are actually black, the others being brown and gray. The female spider is the larger of the sexes, often measuring 1 to 1.5 cm long, with a leg span of 4 to 5 cm. The female has a unique hourglass mark, usually red, on the ventral abdominal surface. Newly hatched spiders are almost entirely red, darkening with progressive molts. Males are 3 to 5 mm long, with white stripes along the lateral aspect of the abdomen.

Only adult females can envenomate. The bite usually feels like a mild pinprick (and may not be noticed), with subsequent slight redness that usually disappears within a few minutes to an hour. Systemic symptoms of envenomation begin ten to sixty minutes after the bite of the female and are caused by the release of the neurotransmitters acetylcholine and norepinephrine. A few minutes after the bite, a small wheal appears, followed within fifteen to sixty minutes, in a minority of cases, by a band of excruciating cramping pain that remains localized or spreads to involve the thigh, shoulder, back, and abdominal muscles. A boardlike abdomen often simulates an acute abdomen. Bites on the arm can produce chest pain that mimics a myocardial infarction. Hypertension, respiratory distress, seizures, and, occasionally in the very young or old, cardiopulmonary arrest are all possible complications. These symptoms frequently subside in twenty-four hours, but in a few cases recur for several days to months. The very young, very old, and those with hypertension have the greatest risk of morbidity from *Latrodectus* envenomation.

Reassure the patient and have him or her rest as much as possible. Assess ABCs and monitor vital signs. Attempt to assess whether the individual was indeed bitten by a spider or whether another process is occurring. Cold applied to the bite site may reduce localized pain somewhat. If significant pain is present, immobilize the involved extremity. Pressure immobilization with elastic bandage is not recommended as retention of venom at the bite site increases local symptoms (reference: Couser, G.A., and G.J.Wilkes. 1997. A red-back spider bite in a lymphoedematous arm. *Med J Aust* 166:587–88). Oral analgesics are useful for muscle pain.

If available, narcotics may be necessary for pain control, but care must be taken to avoid hypotension and respiratory depression. A number of therapies for *Latrodectus* envenomation (such as muscle relaxants and IV calcium gluconate) have been tried with limited success (Category 2). Diazepam should be administered with caution to an intoxicated victim as this potentiates CNS depression. There is little doubt that antivenin is the most effective therapy; however, the safety of the IV antivenin used in North America is of concern. In Australia and Japan, a different antivenin is used IM with an excellent safety and efficacy record. Due to the difficulties of storing antivenin, its field use cannot be recommended. Immediate evacuation is recommended for signs of serious envenomation.

2. Fiddleback

While often called brown recluses, fiddlebacks are not always distinctively brown. They most often have a distinctive violin or fiddle-shaped mark on the dorsal cephalothorax. They average 12 mm long, with a leg span of up to 5 cm. The bite of both sexes is equally venomous, although it's usually painless. Within a few hours, a macule or vesicle may appear at the site. In a severe bite, erythema and blistering follow within six to twelve hours. The classic picture is a hemorrhagic vesicle surrounded by a white or pale ischemic zone, and then by an erythematous region—the so-called bull's-eye lesion. By inspection of the lesion alone, however, it is usually impossible to differentiate a *Loxosceles* bite from many other skin lesions and bites. Pruritus and rash can also occur. Nausea, vomiting, headache, and fever are common systemic symptoms. The lesion either resolves or becomes necrotic and indurated. This may require excision or grafting. Symptoms of envenomation with fiddleback bites are caused by cell and tissue injury and direct lytic action of sphingomyelinase on red cell membranes. Rarely, and mostly in children, massive intravascular hemolysis develops early, often before the local necrotic lesion is well established. If the systemic symptoms include pallor and bloody urine, urgent evacuation is indicated (reference: Pitts, R. M., M. Callahan, E. Owings, and W. King. 1992. Tough spiders: Identifying and treating their bites. In *The Children's Hospital of Alabama poison information bulletin,* Vol. 21, No. 1, Southeast Child Safety Institute).

Treatment consists of local wound care. If the wound becomes necrotic and extends to more than 1 cm in diameter, the use of oral dapsone may be indicated (Category 2). Do not use dapsone unless the person has been tested for G6P deficiency. The short-term application of ice packs to the bite site is as effective as any other form of therapy. The patient may be placed on a corticosteroid, such as prednisone 1 mg/kg daily for five days, during the acute phase.

C. Scorpion stings

Approximately 650 species of scorpions inhabit the world, mainly distributed in tropical and subtropical areas. An estimated forty of these species live in the United States, distributed across 75 percent of the country but concentrated in the warmer regions. All scorpions inject venom through a single sharp stinger at the tip of the "tail," which is actually an extension of the abdomen.

Contact with scorpions is usually accidental. They feed at night. During the daytime they may take shelter in clothing, boots, and bedding. Outdoors, they may often be found under rocks and logs. Checking their hiding places in known scorpion areas is good advice for any traveler. Although the sting is painful, few species inject sufficient venom to be of concern to humans. The only potentially lethal U.S. scorpion is *Centruroides exilicauda* (or *sculpturatus*). *C. gertschi* is generally considered a variety of sculpturatus. This scorpion is found in the Southwest, primarily in Arizona. It is most active May through August, hibernating in winter. Since specific identification is difficult, the traveler is advised to inquire locally about what dangerous species are present before traveling into scorpion territory. As with black widow spiders, most deaths and serious reactions from *Centruroides* stings are in small children, the elderly, and hypertensives.

Any sting typically produces a burning pain, minimal swelling, redness, vesicles, numbness, tingling, and, uncommonly, weakness or numbness of the affected extremity. *Centruroides* stings are usually acutely painful, with a hypersensitive zone soon developing around the site. The injured area may be sensitive to touch, pressure, heat, and cold. Salivation, diaphoresis, perioral paresthesias, dysphagia, gastric distention, hyperactivity, diplopia, nystagmus, visual loss, incontinence, penile erection, exaggerated reflexes, abdominal pain, opisthotonos, seizures, hypertension (more common), hypotension (less common), pulmonary edema, coma, and muscle paralysis (including respiratory paralysis) can ensue, especially in children. Most nonlethal symptoms last less than four hours.

Treatment includes evaluation and application of cold to the sting site. Clean the site and apply a sterile, or at least clean, dressing. For severe pain, splint or immobilize the affected extremity. Oral, nonnarcotic analgesics may be useful. If serious symptoms develop (see those listed in the previous paragraph), immediate evacuation is indicated. If possible, bring the scorpion along on the evacuation, but avoid direct handling.

For those with the skill and equipment, benzodiazepine or phenobarbital may be used for seizures and excitability. Methocarbamol may be administered IV for severe muscle spasms. Oral or parenteral antihypertensive medications (such as clonidine) may be required. If there are profound cholinergic effects, administer atropine. Give IV fluids carefully, if needed, since pulmonary edema may develop. Observe all healthy adults for at least four hours after a sting. Admit to the hospital all children and elderly patients stung by scorpions.

Administer IV antivenin only in cases of severe poisoning. It is available in most areas where dangerous scorpions exist. In the United States, it is only available in Arizona. Test for sensitivity to the serum only if the antivenin is to be used. Administer tetanus immunization.

D. Centipede bites

Centipedes are found all over the United States. They rarely cause serious injury to humans. The giant desert centipede, which may attain a length of 15 cm (6 inches), can give a painful bite. Most bite reactions are local and no fatalities have been documented, but renal failure has been reported. Generally, centipedes hide in dark places. Check shoes, clothing, and bedding before use while traveling in centipede-infested areas.

Local reactions to centipede bites, in addition to intense pain, may include edema and erythema, lasting four to twelve hours. In severe bites, tenderness may persist or recur. To prevent secondary infection, cleanse the wound with soap and water. Apply cold and/or give oral analgesics for pain. In more serious reactions, where there is local lymphangitis, evidence of local necrosis at the bite site, or the rare systemic reaction, evacuate the patient. In case there is severe pain, infiltrate locally with lidocaine.

For centipede bites, observe patients with minor reactions for approximately four hours, or until the reaction improves. Admit patients with evidence of significant reaction because of potential rhabdomyolysis and acute renal failure. Tetanus prophylaxis should be current.

Millipedes do not bite, but they may have secretions that irritate the skin. Treat by washing with soap and water (not alcohol) and applying a corticosteroid cream or lotion.

E. Tetanus immunization

Because of the possibility of contaminated skin, tetanus immunization should be current for all bites and stings, regardless of the species inflicting the injury.

22

Tick-Transmitted Diseases

Recommendations are considered Category 1A, except where indicated 2, by the WMS Panel of Expert Reviewers.

I. GENERAL INFORMATION

Ticks are vectors of many serious infections, more than any other North American arthropod, although in number of infections, mosquitoes spreading West Nile virus are surpassing them. The more common infections transmitted by hard ticks (Ixodidae) include Lyme disease and Southern tick-associated rash illness (STARI), Rocky Mountain spotted fever, ehrlichiosis, babesiosis, tularemia, and Colorado tick fever. These ticks also cause tick paralysis, a noninfectious disorder. Soft ticks (Argasidae) are vectors of relapsing fever.

Several measures lessen the likelihood of being bitten by a tick or acquiring a tickborne illness. Light-colored clothing allows ticks to be more easily seen. Long-sleeved shirts and long pants, particularly with trousers tucked inside high socks, help keep ticks away. Contact with brush should be avoided, if possible.

Permethrin applied to clothing kills ticks so effectively that it appears to repel them. A repellent containing DEET, which is essentially entirely safe when used as directed, may be applied to exposed skin. A concentration of DEET no greater than 30 percent is recommended, and it has recently been approved for children older than two months by the American Academy of Pediatrics. Microencapsulated and polymerized preparations remain on the skin longer, and less of them is absorbed.

Close examination, preferably unclothed, is a significant element of tick avoidance, but it is not practical with youth groups, where reliance on the prevention of tick bites by the protective effects of permethrin-treated clothing is preferable. Examination once every twenty-four hours is sufficient because hard ticks require more time to become attached and transmit infections. These ticks may not attach for several hours after initial skin contact and can be easily removed. Showering or bathing may remove unattached ticks. Once attached, tick removal is more difficult, but the tick must be removed without delay.

The most widely recommended method of tick removal is to grasp it as close as possible to the point of attachment with sharp-pointed tweezers, and pull gently. The mouthparts may not be removed with the rest of the tick but are usually extruded later, although they may become infected. Remaining mouthparts do not transmit infections. Do not crush the tick. Clean the wound with soap and water and disinfect the tweezers. More efficient than using sharp-pointed tweezers is to use any of three commercial tick-removal tools: the Original Tickked Off, the Pro-Tick Remedy, and the Tick Plier, also called the Tick Nipper. (References: Hayes, E. B., and J. Piesman. 2003. How can we prevent Lyme disease? *New Eng J Med* 348:2,424–30. Stewart, R. L., W. Burgdorfer, and G. R. Needham. 1998. Evaluation of three commercial tick removal tools. *JWEM* 9:137–42.)

II. GUIDELINES FOR ASSESSMENT AND TREATMENT

A. Lyme disease

Lyme disease is a worldwide, tickborne infection caused by *Borrelia* spirochetes. In the United States, areas of high risk are the Northeast, the upper Midwest, California, southern Oregon, and western Nevada. The organism is spread by deer ticks (*Ixodes scapularais*) in the Northeast and Midwest and by *I. pacificus* on the West Coast. Most infections occur between May 1 and November 30.

The first sign is usually an expanding circular red rash (erythema chronicum migrans) that occurs at the site where the tick was attached. Flulike symptoms often develop with the rash.

In individuals who are not treated, disseminated infection, manifested by multiple annular secondary rashes, neurologic abnormalities (meningitis, Bell's palsy, peripheral neuropathy), arthralgias, and heart involvement (most commonly atrioventricular block) may appear several weeks after the tick bite. Months after an untreated infection, arthritis may develop, usually affecting the knees and shoulders. Persistent and varied neurologic abnormalities may occur and persist for years.

Early treatment shortens the duration of erythema migrans and diminishes the likelihood of secondary and tertiary sequelae. Doxycycline for fourteen to twenty-one days is recommended for localized and early disseminated infections, except in pregnant women and children eight years old and younger, who should receive amoxicillin. An effective, but expensive, vaccine for Lyme disease has been developed, but it was removed from the market by the manufacturer in February 2002 because sales were low (reference: Steere, A. C. 2001. Lyme disease. *New Eng J Med* 345:115–25).

B. Southern tick-associated rash illness (STARI)

STARI is characterized by a rash essentially identical to erythema migrans, but the rash clears without treatment, and no further symptoms develop. This infection appears to be caused by another species of *Borrelia,* although the organism has not been cultured. It is transmitted by lone star ticks *Amblyomma americanum* and is limited to the Southeastern states where that tick is found.

C. Rocky Mountain spotted fever

In spite of its name, 90 percent of Rocky Mountain spotted fever (RMSF) infections occur along the east coast of the United States, although infections do occur in all forty-eight contiguous states except Maine. The infection is spread by a number of Ixodes ticks, most commonly the wood tick (*Dermacentor andersoni*) and the dog tick (*Dermacentor variabilis*). The domestic dog is the major host.

Two to fourteen days after a bite by an infected tick, mild chilliness, loss of appetite, and malaise appear. Chills, fever, bone and muscle pain, severe headache, and confusion follow these mild symptoms. Abdominal pain, joint pain, and diarrhea may be present. The triad of fever, severe headache, and rash occurring in the spring, summer, or fall should suggest rickettsial infection. Diagnosis is aided by a history of a tick bite in an endemic area.

Younger patients usually develop the rash earlier. Most often small, flat, pink, nonpruritic macules, which blanch when pressure is applied, first appear on the wrists, forearms, and ankles. Eventually the lesions become raised and spread over the entire body, frequently including the palms and soles. However, the characteristic petechial rash is usually not seen until the sixth day or later after the onset of symptoms, and this rash occurs in only 35 to 60 percent of infected individuals. This rash is caused by hemorrhages into the skin from infected, inflamed blood vessels. In severe cases, blotchy red areas appear all over the body, and the individuals appear seriously ill.

RMSF can be a very severe illness, and patients often require hospitalization. The organisms infect endothelial cells throughout the body and may involve the respiratory system, central nervous system, gastrointestinal system, or renal system. Untreated infections last about two weeks and have a mortality of 20 to 30 percent; treatment reduces mortality to 3 to 10 percent. Severe or fatal infections are associated with advanced age, male sex, African-American race, chronic alcohol abuse, and glucose-6-phosphate dehydrogenase (G-6-PD) deficiency.

Initiate appropriate antibiotic treatment immediately on the basis of clinical and epidemiologic findings whenever Rocky Mountain spotted fever is suspected. Treatment must not be delayed until laboratory confirmation is obtained. If the patient is treated within the first four or five days, fever generally subsides within twenty-four to seventy-two hours. Failure to respond to a tetracycline antibiotic argues against a diagnosis of RMSF.

Preventive therapy in individuals who have had recent tick bites is not recommended and may, in fact, only delay the onset of disease.

D. Ehrlichiosis

The ehrlichia are obligate intracellular bacteria that infect a variety of animals and are usually vectored by ticks. Infection in humans, which was first recognized in the United States in 1986, takes two forms: human monocytic ehrlichiosis (HME), in which morules are formed in peripheral blood monocytes; and human granulocytic ehrlichiosis (HGE), in which morules are formed in peripheral blood granulocytes.

Most HGE infections have occurred in the north-central United States (e.g., Minnesota and Wisconsin) and in the New England area (e.g., Connecticut and New York). The same Ixodes ticks that vector Lyme disease and babesiosis, *I. scapularis* in the northeastern United States and *I. pacificus* in the western coastal United States, transmit the agent.

HME is transmitted to humans by the bite of the lone star tick, *Amblyomma americanum.* The wood tick, *D. variabilis,* has also been implicated. Reported infections are concentrated in the the south-central states of Arkansas, Missouri, Oklahoma, and eastern Texas, and in North Carolina and Virginia.

The clinical courses of infections by either organism are quite similar. Typically the first manifestation is an acute febrile illness associated with headache and myalgia. Approximately 75 percent of patients have a history of tick exposure. Laboratory studies usually disclose leukopenia and thrombocytopenia, sometimes anemia, and elevated hepatic aminotransferases. A nonspecific rash occurs in approximately one-third of the patients with HME, but it is less common in patients with HGE.

The diagnosis is aided by finding organisms in peripheral blood smears, but typical morules are found in only about 80 percent of serologically confirmed infections. Infections are most often diagnosed or confirmed by immunofluorescence assay (IFA), although polymerase chain reaction (PCR) assays are being used more commonly.

Most patients have a mild illness that rapidly responds to doxycycline (100 mg twice a day). Defervesence usually occurs in twenty-four to forty-eight hours. However, a significant number of individuals, mostly older patients, have life-threatening complications that include adult respiratory distress syndrome (ARDS), renal failure, neurologic disorders, and disseminated intravascular coagulation (DIC). Case-fatality ratios as high as 10 percent for HGE and 5 percent for HME have been reported, but these appear high (reference:

McQuiston, J. H., C. D. Paddock, R. C. Holman, et al. The human ehrli-chioses in the United States. *Emerging Infectious Diseases.* www.cdc.gov/ncidod/eid/vol5no5/mcquiston.htm [accessed May 8, 2005]).

E. Babesiosis

Babesiosis is an infection by intraerythrocytic Babesia parasites. In the north-eastern United States it has the same distribution as Lyme disease. The main etiologic agent is *B. microti,* and it is transmitted by the same tick, *I. scapularis,* and has the same principal animal reservoir, the white-footed mouse, *Peromyscus leucopus.* A second pattern includes cases reported from California, Georgia, and Washington, but the etiologic agents have not been speciated.

Clinical signs of infection vary considerably; many patients remain asymp-tomatic. Symptoms are similar to malaria, also an intraerythrocytic parasite, except the periodicity of malaria is not seen. Symptoms usually appear one to four weeks following a tick bite and consist of the gradual onset of malaise, anorexia, and fatigue. Within a week or so, a fever that ranges from 100° to 104°F (37.8° to 40.3°C), drenching sweats, and myalgia develop. As with malaria, nausea, vomiting, headache, shaking chills, hemoglobinuria, altered mental status, disseminated intravascular coagulation, anemia with dyserythropoiesis, hypotension, respiratory distress, and renal insufficiency are common.

Severe and fatal cases of human babesiosis occur most commonly in eld-erly patients, patients who have had a splenectomy, and patients who are immuno-deficient. In spleen-intact patients, parasitemia usually ranges from 1 to 20 percent, although parasitemia of 85 percent has been reported. Hemolytic ane-mia and thrombocytopenia are frequent, and the urine may be dark.

Examination of blood smears has been the most useful diagnostic proce-dure. The tetrad (Maltese-cross) forms of the parasite are typical, although the predominant forms in most blood smears closely resemble the rings of Plas-modia. Difficulty in distinguishing between the two organisms is avoided primarily because their ranges do not appear to overlap. An indirect immuno-fluorescent antibody assay (IFA) is available.

Quinine combined with clindamycin is the treatment of choice.

F. Infections with multiple organisms

The first reported fatal case of Lyme disease occurred in a patient who also had babesiosis. In a study from Block Island, Rhode Island, sixteen of forty-six sub-jects with babesiosis also had *B. burgdorfor* infections. In a study of 240 Long Island and Connecticut patients with Lyme disease, twenty-six (11 percent) also had babesiosis. Coinfected patients had a greater incidence of fatigue, headache, sweats, chills, anorexia, emotional lability, nausea, conjunctivitis, and splenomegaly. Half of the coinfected patients were symptomatic for three months or longer, but only seven (4 percent) of 184 patients with Lyme dis-ease alone (and available for follow-up) had illnesses that persisted that long.

Coinfected patients also experienced more symptoms and a more persistent illness than those with babesiosis alone.

Investigators who studied adult *I. scapularis* ticks from Wisconsin, Massachusetts (Nantucket Island), and New York (Westchester County), collected between 1982 and 1995, found that between 2.2 percent and 26 percent were coinfected with *B. burgdorferi* and an agent resembling *Ehrlichia equi,* the cause of HGE. Simultaneous infections with two or even three of these organisms should be anticipated.

G. Tularemia

Humans are highly susceptible to infection with the organism, which occurs most often through the bite of an arthropod. Ticks are the most common vector in the United States, particularly in the central and Rocky Mountain states, where most infections occur. (Biting flies are responsible for many infections in California, Nevada, and Utah.) The most commonly infected ticks are the lone star tick (*A. americanum*), the dog tick (*D. variabilis*), and the wood tick (*D. andersoni*).

After the bite of an infected arthropod, the incubation period averages about three to five days, but the range is one to twenty-one days. After cutaneous inoculation, *Francisella tularensis* multiplies at the local site and produces a papule. Ulceration follows two to four days later. At this point, organisms spread locally to regional lymph nodes and then may disseminate through the blood and lymphatics.

Six classic forms of the disease have been described—ulceroglandular, glandular, oculoglandular, oropharyngeal, typhoidal, and pneumonic—based on clinical presentation of the illness. These forms frequently overlap in individual patients.

The treatment of choice for tularemia has been streptomycin, but recent shortages of this drug have forced reliance on other agents. Prospective, controlled data about these drugs do not exist. Gentamicin at a dosage of 5.4 to 7.5 mg/kg a day intravenously in divided doses every eight hours (mean, 6 mg/kg a day) for seven to fourteen days, depending upon clinical response, has been effective. Tetracycline and its derivatives have been shown to be effective, but they are generally reserved for less severe infections.

H. Colorado tick fever

Colorado tick fever is the most common human arbovirus infection. It is transmitted exclusively by female wood ticks (*D. andersoni*) in North America, and its distribution roughly approximates that of this vector. The virus has been isolated from humans and from ticks in California, Colorado, Idaho, Montana, Nevada, New Mexico, Oregon, South Dakota, Utah, Washington, and Wyoming, and also in Canada's southern Alberta and British Columbia. This infection continues to be underrecognized and underreported.

People with recreational or occupational exposure to ticks in the period April through June have a higher incidence of infection. After an incubation period of less than one to nineteen days (average, about four days), the onset is usually abrupt and is characterized by high fever, chills, joint and muscle pains, severe headache, ocular pain, conjunctival injection, nausea, and occasional vomiting. The spleen and liver may be palpable. A transitory petechial or maculopapular rash is seen in a few individuals.

No specific signs or symptoms, physical findings, or laboratory abnormalities define Colorado tick fever, but the diagnosis is strongly suggested if the illness is interrupted by an afebrile, symptom-free interval that lasts two to three days. Fifty percent of the individuals with clinical illness manifest this interval.

Colorado tick fever is rarely a life-threatening illness, but it can cause severe discomfort, and symptoms may last for some weeks. A few individuals have a more severe illness that produces extended prostration, anorexia, continuing fatigue, and convalescence for several more weeks. Children may have hemorrhagic manifestations ranging from a more pronounced rash to disseminated intravascular coagulopathy and gastrointestinal bleeding.

The diagnosis is confirmed by serologic testing. No specific therapy or vaccine is available.

I. Tick paralysis

Tick paralysis has been recognized since 1912 and involves humans and animals. This disorder is found worldwide, but it occurs most often in North America and Australia. The Pacific Northwest and Rocky Mountain areas account for most cases. At least forty-three species of tick have been reported to cause tick paralysis, but the dog tick, *D. variabilis,* and the wood tick, *D. andersoni,* are the most common vectors.

Tick paralysis occurs during the spring and summer when ticks are feeding. Children are affected more often than adults, and girls are affected twice as often as boys, possibly because their long hair hides the tick. Men are affected more often than women, probably because they participate in activities that bring them into contact with ticks more frequently.

Tick paralysis is thought to be caused by unidentified venom secreted by the tick salivary glands during a blood meal. The disorder first appears five to six days after attachment of the tick. The earliest symptoms are restlessness, irritability, and paresthesias in the hands and feet. Twenty-four to forty-eight hours later, an ascending, symmetric, flaccid paralysis with loss of deep tendon reflexes appears. Weakness typically is initially worse in the lower extremities.

Within one to two days, severe generalized weakness develops. Cerebellar dysfunction with ataxia and loss of coordination may appear. Dysfunction may progress to bulbar and respiratory paralysis. Isolated facial paralysis may occur in individuals with ticks imbedded behind the ear.

The paralysis resolves after removal of the tick, which establishes the diagnosis. In North America recovery is usually rapid. It starts within hours and is complete within days. Other than removing the tick, no therapy other than supportive care is needed or available. However, undiagnosed tick paralysis can be lethal.

J. Relapsing fever

Relapsing fever is the only major tick infection in the United States transmitted by soft ticks, Argasidae, which are rarely seen, resemble raisins, and may not be recognized as ticks. Unlike Ixodes ticks, the soft *Ornithodoros* ticks rarely remain attached for more than thirty minutes, and the tick bite is often unrecognized.

Hosts for these ticks are wild rodents, and the ticks live in the host's nests or burrows, particularly cracks and crevices in the walls of cabins, and behave like bedbugs. In the United States infections occur primarily in Oregon, Washington, and northern California, although occasional infections occur in other western states. Relapsing fever has a worldwide distribution.

Relapsing fever is caused by *Borrelia* spirochetes and is characterized by bouts of fever that alternate with afebrile periods. The onset is usually sudden and is characterized by fever that commonly is higher than 102.2°F (39°C). Often shaking chills, severe headache, myalgias, arthralgias, nausea and vomiting, muscular weakness, and lethargy accompany the fever and may be associated with sweats and intense thirst. A transitory petechial rash is common during the initial attack. In some cases, meningeal inflammation and peripheral facial palsy have occurred.

An average of six to seven days later, but with a considerable range, the fever reappears. Three relapses is the average, but as many as ten or more can occur. The relapses tend to be progressively less severe. The relapsing nature of this illness appears to be related to antigenic variation. As an immune response develops to the predominant spirochetal antigenic strain, variant strains multiply and cause a recrudescent infection.

The diagnosis is established by identification of the organism in blood smears. Tetracycline and erythromycin are effective antibiotics. To prevent infection, rodent-infested cabins should be avoided.

III. CONTROVERSIES

The two major controversies about tickborne infections are related to Lyme disease. The first concerns prophylactic therapy following a tick bite in high-risk areas. Such therapy would not be necessary unless the tick is attached and is distended with blood. The infection is not transmitted until ticks have been attached for thirty-six hours or more. A single 200 mg dose of doxycycline has been recommended following the finding of a distended tick, and it has the additional benefit of being effective for ehrlichiosis, but even this treatment is controversial.

The second controversy concerns whether chronic Lyme disease exists and how it should be treated. A number of patients with Lyme disease develop persistent complaints that are nonspecific and include arthralgias, myalgias, cognitive difficulties, fatigue, malaise, dizziness, stiff neck, and photophobia. Some patients are severely disabled. Such persistent disability is not uncommon and occurs most frequently in individuals who have not been treated in the early stages of their infection. In some the treatment has been delayed for as long as a year. The entire problem is further confused by a respected study that found the frequency of symptoms of pain and fatigue was no greater in patients who had experienced Lyme disease than in age-matched individuals who had not had this infection.

Klempner and his colleagues were able to find 129 patients (78 with IgG antibodies to *B. burgdorferi* and 51 without) for a study of the effectiveness of antibiotic therapy. They found no difference between treated individuals and controls that received only placebo.

Does chronic Lyme disease really exist? If so, how should it be treated? At the present time no definite answer can be given to the first question, which precludes an answer to the second.

23

Substance Abuse
in Wilderness Settings

Recommendations are considered Category 2 by the WMS Panel of Expert Reviewers.

I. GENERAL INFORMATION

Although data are sparse, it has been suggested that alcohol places a person at risk for injury or death, particularly in wilderness areas close to roads. Data on the involvement of alcohol and nonprescribed or nonmedically indicated use of mood- and mind-altering chemicals on trauma in wilderness areas is sparse, and it is difficult to draw conclusions. However, the involvement of drug and alcohol misuse is a well-known contributor to trauma outside the wilderness. Parishioners should be aware of this and be alert for acute or chronic intoxication, accidental overdoses, and withdrawal in patients in wilderness settings.

II. GUIDELINES FOR ASSESSMENT AND TREATMENT

In any individual with an illness or injury in the wilderness, mind- or mood-altering drugs may complicate assessment and treatment. Consideration must be given to whether the patient's senses are so altered as to be unaware of his or her true physical state, including the presence of pain or imminent danger. If substance abuse is suspected, take extra time to assess the patient and give additional consideration to stabilization and care.

Working with people who are under the influence of drugs (including ethanol) is often difficult because such individuals may have radical alterations in personality, rapid mood swings, and irrational behavior patterns. A calm, unhurried, yet authoritative approach, especially with the use of a friend of the patient, can be effective in gaining the patient's confidence (or at least the patient's ear) and having him/her acquiesce to treatment.

In addition, advanced providers may have two other modalities: antidotes and sedation. Naloxone (0.4 to 4 mg IV, SQ), if available, will reverse the effects of narcotics and narcotic analogues. Sedation with antipsychotics (haloperidol, chlor-promazine) or benzodiazepines (diazepam, lorazepam) can be used if patients are in danger of harming themselves or others. Extreme care must be exercised to avoid depressing the respiratory drive in such individuals.

24

Anxiety and Stress Reactions in the Wilderness

Recommendations are considered Category 1B by the WMS Panel of Expert Reviewers.

I. GENERAL INFORMATION

Accidental injuries in the wilderness, particularly when severe, are accompanied by significant psychological distress in victims, other party members, and in rescuers. Panic and anxiety reactions are common in stressful situations. Other emotions, such as grief or depression, may also occur. The reactions of victims or witnesses may be so severe that their safety and that of other party members is compromised.

The incidents that generate strong emotions include serious injury or death of a participant or bystander, multiple deaths or serious injuries, serious injury or death of a child, and incidents that attract unusual attention by the media. Having a person die in spite of diligent rescue efforts and intensive care is particularly stressful. An immediate stress reaction is normal, not a sign of psychological problems, and may have physical, emotional, cognitive, and behavioral components.

II. CARE IN THE FIELD

Medical care for physical injuries, and securing the safety of all party members, should take first priority following a wilderness accident. But care for anxiety and stress reactions, which should be anticipated, can begin almost immediately, and it should be given regardless of whether the individual is manifesting signs or symptoms. Some basic considerations in anxiety management include the following:

- Injured persons should be encouraged to talk. They can talk about anything and may ramble about totally unrelated events. Gentle encouragement to talk about how they are feeling at the moment is helpful.
- The primary role of the psychologic caregiver is to listen and show concern.
- Realistic, but optimistic, feedback should be provided. Questions must be answered truthfully, but gently.
- Injured persons should be encouraged, even pushed, to play as large a role in their care and rescue as possible to help restore their self-esteem and sense of self-worth.

III. MEDICATIONS

Drugs should be avoided if possible, but when needed, the drugs of choice for anxiety reduction are the benzodiazepines: diazepam (Valium), chlordiazepoxide (Librium), and alprazolam (Xanax). Although other drugs, such as alcohol, barbiturates, and narcotic analgesics, provide some relief of anxiety, the benzodiazepines are much safer. The primary side effect is mild sedation, and, apart from potential interactions with other sedatives, very few contraindications exist. Therapeutic onset for anxiety relief takes one to three hours with typical oral dosages. Diazepam is the fastest. Haldol, 5 to 10 mg intramuscularly or orally, is also effective.

IV. CARE FOR RESCUERS

Rescuers must mask their emotions in order to perform well during the rescue. Failure to relieve such pent-up emotions can lead to psychologic problems, particularly posttraumatic stress disorder (PTSD). One proven way to reduce or eliminate such problems is a group discussion, usually held after physical recovery, to discuss feelings during the rescue. The session must be limited to that topic; the rescue must be critiqued at another time. The discussion must be entirely nonjudgmental and include only a discussion of what was actually felt. Obviously no feelings that actually were experienced can be right or wrong. Professional guidance may be desirable after a particularly stressful event.

V. REFERRAL AND FOLLOW-UP

Victims of traumatic events, like their rescuers, are at increased risk of developing PTSD and should be told about symptoms that signify the need for additional treatment. Primary symptoms of PTSD include distressing dreams or reliving the trauma; persistent avoidance, psychogenic amnesia, or numbing in response to trauma-related stimuli; and increased somatic nervous system arousal or hypervigilance. Any or all of these symptoms are part of the normal human reaction to trauma, but their persistence beyond a month is indicative of PTSD.

Clinical psychologists and psychiatrists who specialize in anxiety and stress disorders have developed effective treatments for this disorder. Cognitive-behavioral therapies and certain drugs have proven effective, alone and in combinations.

VI. OTHER CONSIDERATIONS

Emotional and behavioral disorders are common; incidence rates in the general adult population are 10 percent for anxiety disorders, 6 percent for major depression, and at least 5 percent for personality disorders. Although wilderness adventurers may be robust and seem resistant to emotional distress, some outing members develop psychological problems. Most people undergo emotional changes in harsh environments, and personal conflicts add stress to group dynamics. The success of a wilderness expedition depends significantly on the "people skills" of the leaders.

25

Wilderness Medical Kits

Recommendations are considered Category 1B by the WMS Panel of Expert Reviewers.

I. GENERAL INFORMATION

Preparations for wilderness activities include provisions for emergency care of individuals in the event of injuries or illnesses. Trip medical leaders must be able to assemble medical kits that are appropriate to support the proposed trip. This requires assessing several factors.

A. Purpose of the trip

Selectivity is the key in choosing appropriate medical equipment. Groups intent only on providing self-treatment should consider the most common injuries they will sustain. Because a search and rescue (SAR) team must be equipped to handle the medical emergencies that they expect to encounter, they can justify carrying specialized medical gear. On recreational trips, however, the medical kit displaces other equipment that might be needed. Hikers, whitewater enthusiasts, and climbers all need different medical kits to meet their specialized needs.

B. Level of medical training

It may be inappropriate to include medications and equipment that no trip member has the requisite knowledge or experience to use safely. Trip members responsible for medical care of the group should have direct input into the contents of the medical kit. Levels of training and experience can differ widely among groups of physicians, nurses, and EMS personnel. A degree or license may not guarantee knowledge in any specific area. Pretrip training to supplement the knowledge base of the providers may be advisable.

C. Destination

The terrain, altitude, weather, propensity for endemic diseases, and other inherent dangers must be considered. Groups heading into remote areas where local inhabitants may request medical help must consider this potential demand on their supplies, and they must consider whether they intend to respond.

D. Length of trip

The total time that the party must be supported from the kit affects its contents. Some problems are likely to occur only during particular times. For example, the treatment of friction blisters is most important during the first few days of a hike. At times on a long trip, outside medical supplies can be obtained to restock the kit.

E. Time for evacuation or medical rescue

Some trips progressively distance themselves from medical care. On other trips, time required to obtain help may be deceptive. A river-raft trip into a canyon, for instance, may last only hours, but evacuation in the event of an accident may take many days of dangerous and laborious effort.

F. Size of the party

Although an increase in the number of participants influences the quantity of some medications and bandaging materials, the increase is not linear. Frequently, only minimal additions are needed to serve a larger group adequately. Equipping each member with a personal kit containing bandages, blister supplies, and personal medications can reduce the size of the main medical kit for a large party.

G. Bulk, weight, and cost

Even if cost is not a consideration, the weight and bulk of a kit are potential limiting factors. Because bandaging and splints are bulky and possibly awkward to carry, the use of improvised materials, such as clothing for bandaging and local fabrication of splints, may be incorporated into plans for the medical kit. Using multifunctional components may also reduce medical equipment. If one piece of equipment or a drug can be used for many different purposes, weight can be significantly reduced. Knowledgeable medical team members are needed to optimize this tactic.

Some organizations and search and rescue teams use a modular approach to medical kits. Separate kits, with increasing sophistication and for various purposes, are available for individuals and situations requiring more advanced equipment. While the basic kit is designed for use by lay personnel, only specially trained individuals can use the more advanced kits, and they carry them into the field only when required.

II. CONTAINERS

Containers for the medical kit must be chosen for maximal accessibility and protection of contents. Damage is to be expected and may render materials useless. In situations where there is danger of the loss of equipment, such as on white-water trips, the medical kit components should be divided into several kits so that all equipment is not lost if an accident occurs. Individuals with life-sustaining medications should take an extra quantity to be carried separately.

The medical kit must be easily identified and accessible when needed. This entails making it visible (e.g., bright red and/or marked with reflective material) and placing it where it can be reached easily. Kits that unroll or open to display their contents make selection of items very convenient. For small kits this is not usually necessary. For large kits, kits that will be used frequently, and kits that may be accessed by multiple members of the group, accessibility and easy identification of contents are very important.

III. GUIDELINES FOR EQUIPMENT

Equipment for a wilderness medical kit should be selected in light of its function.

A. Life support

Airways, supplemental oxygen, manually powered suction devices, chest tubes, and similar equipment are generally only carried by experienced rescue personnel on prolonged remote expeditions.

B. Vital signs

A watch with a second hand to time pulse or respiration is an important piece of equipment. A blood-pressure cuff and stethoscope are useful in some situations, but they may be of no value to untrained personnel.

C. Soft-tissue injuries

An irrigation syringe will provide adequate wound-cleaning capability. Wound-closure materials range from butterfly bandages and wound-closure strips to suture equipment with surgical instruments or surgical staples. Cleansing materials, local anesthetics, and bandaging materials are also in this category. Material for blister treatment is probably the most commonly used item in this group.

D. Orthopedic injuries

Prefabricated splints are now manufactured in lightweight designs, including collapsible femoral traction splints, but these may be improvised in the field. Cervical collars may likewise be improvised. Backboards or litters are not usually needed, except by rescue groups. Fiberglass casting material makes an excellent lightweight splinting material.

E. Medication administration

Special equipment in addition to the medications is necessary only if injectable drugs or intravenous fluids are carried. Injectable medications are susceptible not only to damage from bottle breakage, but also from light, heat, and cold.

IV. MEDICATIONS

The decision to carry any particular medication must take into account the medical knowledge required to use the medication properly, as well as the cost, bulk, and weight of the kit; the potential problems that may be encountered; medication allergy history of trip participants; and knowledge of local laws and regulations that may restrict possession of certain medications.

A list of potential candidates for inclusion in this list can be obtained by referring to suggestions made in these position papers, various books on wilderness-related medical care, the physician's personal medical/surgical knowledge, and standard texts and publications concerning treatment of trauma and infectious diseases. *The Wilderness Medicine* magazine and *The Journal of Wilderness & Environmental Medicine,* publications of the Wilderness Medical Society, periodically print articles with suggestions for customized medical kits for various remote-area, climatic, and endeavor-specific activities.

26

Immunizations

Recommendations are considered Category 1A by the WMS Panel of Expert Reviewers.

I. GENERAL INFORMATION

Appropriate immunizations are vital for those entering wilderness and foreign areas. Current recommendations for U.S. travelers are issued by the Centers for Disease Control and Prevention (CDC), published annually in *Health Information for International Travel*. The publication contains vaccination and certification requirements for malaria and yellow fever on a country-by-country basis. It also includes the U.S. Public Health Service recommendations for difficult immunization questions, such as immunization of infants and pregnant or lactating women, and specific recommendations for vaccination and prophylaxis for a wide variety of disorders. It also contains a discussion of specific potential health hazards worldwide, grouped by geographic region. The information in this book is updated in the biweekly *Summary of Health Information for International Travel*. Both the book and updates can be obtained from the Superintendent of Documents, U.S. Government Printing Office, Washington, DC 20402. A weekly report of infectious diseases in the United States and important overseas medical developments is contained in the CDC publication *Morbidity and Mortality Weekly Report*. Subscriptions can be obtained from the CDC, Atlanta, GA 30333, or from the Massachusetts Medical Society, C.S.P.O. Box 9120, Waltham, MA 02254-9120, which reprints these reports as part of an inexpensive subscription service.

The United States Centers for Disease Control and Prevention can be accessed via the Internet at www.cdc.gov/travel.

The United States Department of State has a twenty-four-hour hot line that provides general country information, with a travel risk assessment, at (888) 407–4747, or if calling from Canada or from overseas, (317) 472–2328. The United States

Department of State Web site at www.travel.state.gov lists travel warnings and counselor information sheets. Also available on the Internet are travel advisories from the countries of Australia (www.dfat.gov.au/consular/advice), Canada (www.dfait-maeci .gc.ca), and the United Kingdom (www.fco.gov.uk/travel).

An alternative source of information is *Vaccination Certificate Requirements and Health Advice for International Travelers,* published yearly by the World Health Organization, Geneva, Switzerland. It is available through the WHO Publication Center U.S.A., 49 Sheridan Avenue, Albany, NY 12210. Contact the WHO via the Internet at www.who.int.

The local county or state board of health will frequently have information from the abovementioned sources available for consultation and/or will have a referral service to local travel-medicine specialists.

Current immunization advice, disease risk charts, and other information concerning the availability of medical care within foreign countries can be obtained from IAMAT (International Association for Medical Assistance to Travelers), 1623 Military Road #279, Niagara Falls, NY 14304-1745 (716–754–4883) or 40 Regal Road, Guelph, Ontario, Canada N1K 1B5 (519–836–0102). IAMAT provides this information to travelers and physicians free of charge, operating only with donations. Contact IAMAT via the Internet at www.iamat.org.

The Scope of Wilderness Medicine

Our interests include the following areas:

- Physiologic interactions of environmental forces on human performance and health
- Environmental health disorders
  - Heat illness
  - Hypothermia, hyperthermia
  - Frostbite
  - Altitude illness
  - Barotrauma submersion
- Health risks in specific environments
  - Mountains
  - Deserts
  - Jungles
  - Marine
  - Aerospace
  - Subterranean (caves)
- Health risks from plants and animals
  - Toxinology
  - Animal attacks
- Traditional medicine in remote environments
  - Wilderness trauma
  - Medical limitations to wilderness travel
- Travel medicine
- Medical services in wilderness settings
  - Search and rescue
  - Organization of wilderness medical services
  - Expedition medicine
- Infectious diseases from the wilderness and foreign travel
- Liability in wilderness medicine
- Education in wilderness medicine
- Global health issues from environmental depredation

Share Our Members' Sense of Adventure

Our physician and professional members are committed to expanding their knowledge of the prevention, diagnosis, and treatment of wilderness diseases and injuries.

Society members include experts in high-altitude physiology and medical problems from exposure to heat and cold. Others work with astronauts and aquanauts or treat the victims of animal attacks, poisonous bites, and stings. Many WMS members play an integral role in wilderness medical issues within government, civic, and medical organizations.

Wilderness Medical Society Mission Statement

Mission
To advance health care, research, and education related to wilderness medicine.

Philosophy
Founded in 1983, the Wilderness Medical Society (WMS) is the world's leading organization devoted to wilderness medical challenges. Wilderness medicine topics include expedition and disaster medicine, dive medicine, search and rescue, altitude illness, cold- and heat-related illness, wilderness trauma, and wild-animal attacks. The Society explores health risks and safety issues in extreme situations such as mountains, jungles, deserts, caves, marine environments, and space.

Society members have a long-standing commitment to education and research. WMS sponsors accredited continuing medical education conferences that combine exceptional educational presentations with a variety of hands-on workshops. The society publishes a peer-reviewed medical journal, a quarterly newsletter, an educational presentation series, comprised of slides and a text, on wilderness medicine topics, and practice guidelines for wilderness emergency care. Each year the society awards research grants, advancing academic careers and expanding the knowledge and understanding of wilderness medical issues. WMS also fosters Student Interest Groups (SIGs) on seventy-one medical school campuses.

In addition to practicing, investigating, and teaching wilderness medicine, WMS members share a sense of adventure—from exploring deserts to climbing mountains, from scuba diving to white-water rafting, from skiing to windsurfing, from adventure travel to volunteer-relief work. The society's members love the outdoors, have deep respect for the environment and our precious natural resources, and actively support an Environmental Council.

WMS has been classified as a 501(c)3 organization, designating it a charity for public good with a responsibility to educate and serve the public, and indicating that donations may be tax deductible (please consult with a professional tax advisor). To fund the unique WMS programs and publications, the society relies on members (new and renewing), fund-raising events, and charitable gifts and donations. Only with member and public support can the Wilderness Medical Society continue to meet its responsibilities and serve the world beyond its membership.

Join the Wilderness Medical Society today!

Wilderness Medical Society is a one-of-a-kind membership organization where physicians and allied health professionals combine their profession with their passion for wilderness. The society's purpose is to present educational programs and publications that inform its members and the public about preventing, recognizing, and treating medical problems encountered in wilderness situations.

Regular membership in the WMS includes:

- A subscription to *Wilderness and Environmental Medicine,* the official quarterly publication of the Wilderness Medical Society
- A subscription to *Wilderness Medicine,* the society's quarterly newsletter
- Discounts at our online bookstore
- Discounts at our annual meeting
- Eligibility to join the Academy of Wilderness Medicine (see page 124)

Support the society with your financial gift.

The Wilderness Medical Society supports research and environmental preservation with the assistance of generous donors like you.

You can join the WMS or donate at our Web site—www.wms.org—or by phone and post.

WILDERNESS MEDICAL SOCIETY
810 East Tenth Street
Lawrence, KS 66044
Phone: (785) 843–1235, ext. 222

Become a Fellow of the Academy of Wilderness Medicine (FAWM)!

The FAWM program is for health professionals who desire to enhance and demonstrate their knowledge of wilderness and travel medicine.

As FAWM candidates participate in eligible activities, such as the Wilderness Medical Annual Conference, they receive credit toward a preestablished, 100-hour Wilderness Medicine curriculum. The curriculum requires educational experience spread over ninety-four different required topics and many elective topics. The program provides:

- Distinction for professional education in wilderness medicine
- Validation for the public, patients, and clients of training in wilderness medicine
- Recognition for completing high-quality standards in wilderness medicine

The academy's future plans include online learning opportunities, Faculty and Research certifications, and more.

For more information visit our Web site—www.wms.org.

Wilderness Medical Society

810 East Tenth Street
Lawrence, KS 66044
(785) 843–1235, ext. 222
www.wms.org

Joyce Lancaster, WMS Executive Director
Jason Gilbert, WMS Association Manager